Community Health Nursing: Principles, Practices, and Perspectives

Rnda I. Ashgar

Community Health Nursing: Principles, Practices, and Perspectives

A Saudi Approach

Springer

Rnda I. Ashgar
Nursing Department
Jazan University
College of Nursing and Health Sciences
Jazan, Saudi Arabia

ISBN 978-3-032-30790-3 ISBN 978-3-032-30791-0 (eBook)
https://doi.org/10.1007/978-3-032-30791-0

This Springer imprint is published by the registered company Springer Nature Switzerland AG
The registered company address is: Gewerbestrasse 11, 6330 Cham, Switzerland

Dedicated to all nurses who blend science with compassion, tirelessly advocating for their patients and advancing the field of nursing.

Introduction

Community health nursing plays a vital role in enhancing the well-being of populations, particularly in regions where healthcare systems face unique challenges and opportunities. This book delves into the multifaceted nature of community health nursing, focusing specifically on its application within the Saudi Arabian context. It explores the cultural, social, and economic factors that influence healthcare practices and outcomes in Saudi Arabia, offering an in-depth understanding of the strategies employed to address public health concerns in the region. The Saudi healthcare landscape is characterized by a blend of traditional and modern practices, shaped by the country's rapid development and cultural heritage.

This book examines how community health nurses (CHNs) navigate these dynamics to provide effective care. It highlights the importance of culturally competent nursing practices that respect and integrate local customs and beliefs, ensuring that healthcare delivery is both effective and respectful of the community's values. Moreover, the book addresses the specific health issues prevalent in Saudi communities, such as the management of chronic diseases, maternal and child health, and the prevention of communicable diseases. It emphasizes the role of CHNs in promoting health education and awareness, empowering individuals to take charge of their health.

Through a combination of theoretical insights and practical case studies, the book provides readers with a comprehensive overview of community health nursing in Saudi Arabia. It serves as an essential resource for healthcare professionals, educators, and students aiming to understand and contribute to the field of community health nursing in this unique context.

Acknowledgments

I would like to express my heartfelt gratitude to all those who contributed to the development of this book. My deepest thanks go to my colleagues and mentors, whose insights and expertise have been invaluable throughout this journey. I am particularly grateful to my husband and children for their unwavering support and dedication, which helped bring this project to fruition. I would also like to thank the nursing professionals and educators who shared their experiences and knowledge, enriching the content of this book. Your willingness to engage in thoughtful discussions has greatly enhanced the quality of this work. Finally, I wish to acknowledge my family and friends for their patience and encouragement during the writing process. Their belief in me has been a constant source of motivation. Thank you all for your contributions and support.

Contents

About the Author

Dr. Rnda I. Ashgar, PhD, MSN, RN is an Associate Professor of Nursing at Jazan University, Saudi Arabia, specializing in community health nursing and women's health. She earned her Bachelor of Science in Nursing with second honors from King Abdul-Aziz University in 2008 and subsequently received a government scholarship to pursue graduate studies in the United States. She completed her Master of Science in Nursing, majoring in Community Health Nursing, with a GPA of 3.97/4 at Wayne State University in 2013, and later earned her Ph.D. in Nursing Science from the same institution in 2019, achieving a GPA of 3.98/4.

Professionally certified as a Registered Nurse (RN) by the American Board of Nursing in Michigan, Dr. Ashgar is also recognized as a Consultant Community Health Nurse by the Saudi Commission for Health Specialties. Her research primarily focuses on middle-aged women's health, cardiovascular disease risk factors, and health-promoting behaviors.

Dr. Ashgar has held multiple academic and leadership roles at Jazan University, including Dean of the College of Nursing, Vice-Dean for Academic Affairs, and Head of the Nursing Department. She has been actively involved in program development, academic supervision, and national coordination committees for nursing education across Saudi Arabia. She has presented her research at numerous international and national conferences and has authored multiple peer-reviewed publications in journals such as *Journal of Advanced Nursing*, *SAGE Open Nursing*, *The Journal of Cardiovascular Nursing*, and *Nursing Forum*.

Introduction to Community Health Nursing 1

Learning Objectives

By the end of this chapter, students will be able to:

1. Define community health nursing and explain its scope, purpose, and significance within the broader healthcare system.
2. Trace the historical evolution of community health nursing from its public health origins to contemporary practice.
3. Explain how social, economic, and environmental changes have shaped the scope and priorities of community health nursing.
4. Identify and describe the primary roles and responsibilities of community health nurses (CHNs) within diverse community settings.
5. Discuss and apply the core concepts of community health nursing to promote health equity and address social determinants of health.
6. Differentiate among the levels of prevention (primary, secondary, and tertiary) and apply them to community-based disease prevention and health promotion initiatives.
7. Analyze major community health models and frameworks that guide the planning, implementation, and evaluation of public health interventions.
8. Evaluate the importance of interprofessional and intersectoral collaboration, cultural respect, and community participation in improving population health outcomes.
9. Examine current and emerging trends in community health nursing, including technological innovations (telehealth, digital health records), aging populations, and global health challenges.
10. Synthesize knowledge of historical foundations, professional roles, conceptual frameworks, and future trends to design culturally competent, evidence-based strategies that enhance community health and well-being.

R. I. Ashgar, *Community Health Nursing: Principles, Practices, and Perspectives*,
https://doi.org/10.1007/978-3-032-30791-0_1

History and Evolution

Community health nursing is a field deeply rooted in the principles of public health and nursing, evolving significantly over the centuries to meet the changing needs of populations [1]. Initially, the focus was on controlling infectious diseases through sanitation and hygiene practices, which were rudimentary yet essential in reducing mortality rates. The origins of community health nursing can be traced back to the early nineteenth century, when pioneers such as Florence Nightingale began emphasizing the importance of hygiene and sanitary conditions in medical care, particularly during the Crimean War [2, 3]. Her work laid the foundational principles for modern nursing and public health strategies.

As the industrial revolution progressed, urbanization and industrialization brought about new health challenges, including poor living conditions, overcrowding, and pollution, which necessitated a shift in focus from individual patient care to broader public health measures [4]. This period marked the emergence of district nursing in England, where nurses were tasked with providing care to the sick within their homes, a precursor to modern community health nursing practices. The district nursing model emphasized preventive care, health education, and the need for addressing social determinants of health, reflecting a holistic approach to health care, which is still relevant today [5].

In the United States, the establishment of the Henry Street Settlement by Lillian Wald and Mary Brewster in 1893 was a pivotal moment in the history of community health nursing [6]. This initiative aimed to provide accessible healthcare services to the impoverished immigrant populations of New York City's Lower East Side. Wald's work in public health nursing highlighted the necessity of integrating nursing care with social services to address the comprehensive needs of communities, thereby fostering the development of public health nursing as a recognized specialty.

The twentieth century witnessed further evolution in community health nursing, driven by advancements in medical technology and an increasing understanding of epidemiology [7, 8]. The establishment of public health departments and the introduction of systematic disease surveillance and vaccination programs were instrumental in controlling infectious diseases. Community health nurses (CHNs) played a critical role in these efforts, working in collaboration with other health professionals to implement and monitor public health initiatives.

In recent decades, the focus of community health nursing has broadened to include chronic disease management, health promotion, and risk reduction. The rise of noncommunicable diseases, such as diabetes and cardiovascular diseases, has necessitated a shift towards promoting healthy lifestyles and preventive care [9]. CHNs are now integral in designing and implementing health education programs, advocating for policy changes, and conducting research to improve health outcomes at the community level. See Fig. 1.1 for the evolution of community health nursing.

Today, community health nursing continues to evolve in response to global health challenges such as pandemics, environmental changes, and health disparities [1]. The integration of technology, such as telehealth and electronic health records, has

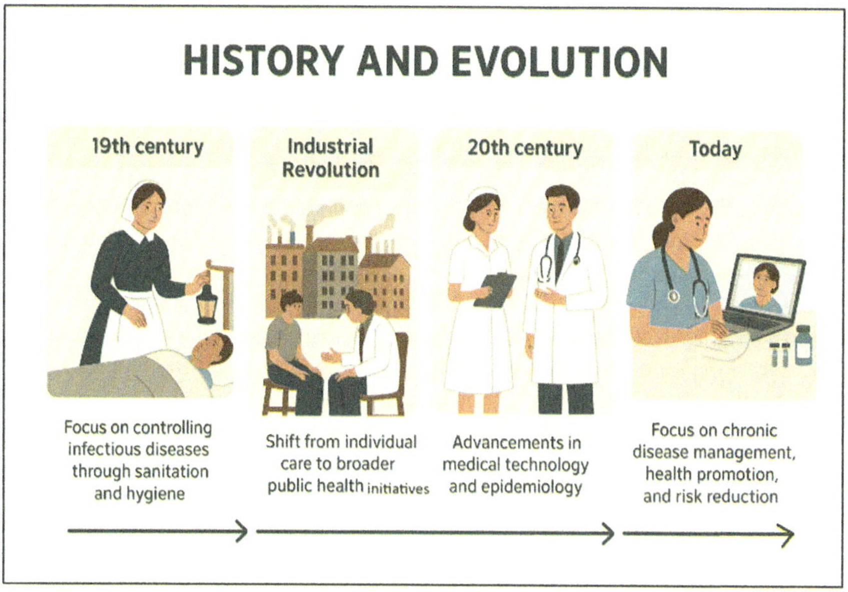

Fig. 1.1 The evolution of community health nursing

enhanced the ability of CHNs to deliver care remotely, expand their reach, and tailor interventions to meet the specific needs of diverse populations. As the field advances, community health nursing remains committed to its core mission of improving the health and well-being of communities through compassionate care, education, and advocacy.

Roles and Responsibilities

Community health nursing plays a pivotal role in bridging the gap between healthcare systems and communities. This domain is characterized by a multifaceted approach where nurses engage with a diverse population, addressing a broad spectrum of health-related issues. The cornerstone of community health nursing lies in its commitment to preventive care, health education, and the promotion of healthy lifestyles among community members. Nurses in this field are not only healthcare providers but also educators, advocates, leaders, and researchers [2, 3, 8].

A primary responsibility of CHNs is to conduct comprehensive community assessments. This involves gathering and analyzing data to identify health needs, resources, and potential barriers to healthcare access within a community. Such assessments enable nurses to devise targeted interventions that address specific health concerns, thereby enhancing the overall well-being of the population. Through these assessments, CHNs can prioritize healthcare initiatives and allocate resources effectively. In addition to assessments, CHNs are tasked with developing and implementing health education programs. These programs are designed to empower individuals and communities with the knowledge and skills necessary for making informed health decisions. By focusing on topics such as nutrition, exercise, disease prevention, and management, nurses help reduce the incidence of chronic illnesses and promote a culture of health consciousness [10].

CHNs also play a critical role in advocating for policies that improve public health. They work collaboratively with policymakers, healthcare providers, and community leaders to influence health policy decisions. By advocating for equitable healthcare access, improved healthcare infrastructure, and the allocation of resources to underserved areas, these nurses strive to eliminate health disparities and foster health equity.

Leadership is another vital aspect of the roles and responsibilities of CHNs. They often coordinate and lead multidisciplinary teams to deliver comprehensive healthcare services. In doing so, they ensure that care is patient-centered and tailored to meet the unique needs of individuals and communities. Leadership in community health nursing also involves mentoring and supporting other healthcare professionals, fostering a collaborative environment that enhances the quality of care. Moreover, CHNs are instrumental in disaster preparedness and response. They develop emergency response plans, conduct training sessions, and engage in simulations to ensure communities are prepared for potential health emergencies. In the event of a disaster, these nurses provide critical support, delivering care to affected individuals and coordinating relief efforts.

The role of CHNs extends to conducting research aimed at improving community health outcomes. By engaging in evidence-based practice, they contribute to the body of knowledge that informs best practices in community health nursing. Through research, they identify effective strategies for disease prevention, health promotion, and the management of health conditions, thereby enhancing the quality of care provided to communities.

In summary, CHNs fulfill a diverse range of roles and responsibilities that are essential to the health and well-being of communities. Through assessment, education, advocacy, leadership, disaster response, and research, they address the multifaceted health needs of populations. Their work is integral to fostering healthier communities and advancing public health objectives.

Core Concepts

In the realm of community health nursing, several core concepts serve as the foundation for practice, guiding nurses in their mission to improve the health and well-being of communities. These concepts are deeply intertwined with the principles of public health and adapted to the unique needs of community settings. Understanding these concepts is essential for any community health nurse aiming to deliver comprehensive and culturally sensitive care. One of the fundamental concepts is the focus on the community as the client. Unlike traditional nursing, which often centers on the individual, community health nursing emphasizes the health of populations and subpopulations.

This approach requires nurses to assess the health status of a community, identify health risks, and develop interventions that address these risks at a community level. By focusing on the community as a whole, nurses can implement strategies that promote health equity and address social determinants of health [11].

Another key concept is the emphasis on prevention. Community health nursing prioritizes primary prevention strategies to avert the onset of disease or injury before it occurs. This proactive approach involves health education, vaccination programs, and advocacy for healthy public policies. Secondary prevention, which focuses on early detection and prompt intervention, and tertiary prevention, aimed at minimizing the impact of chronic illness, also play crucial roles in community health nursing [12].

The principle of partnerships and collaboration is also central to community health nursing. Nurses work alongside community members, local organizations, and other healthcare professionals to identify health priorities and develop appropriate interventions. This collaborative approach ensures that health initiatives are culturally relevant and effectively address the needs of the community. By fostering partnerships, CHNs can leverage resources and expertise to enhance the overall impact of their efforts.

Cultural respect is another vital concept in community health nursing. Nurses must be aware of and sensitive to the cultural beliefs and practices of the communities they serve [13]. This involves not only understanding cultural differences but also respecting and integrating these differences into care delivery. Culturally competent care improves communication, builds trust, and leads to better health outcomes.

Lastly, the concept of empowerment is pivotal in community health nursing. Nurses aim to empower individuals and communities to take control of their health and make informed decisions. This is achieved through education, support, and advocacy, enabling communities to develop self-sufficiency and resilience. Empowerment enhances community capacity to address health issues independently, fostering a sense of ownership and responsibility for health outcomes. These core concepts of community health nursing—community focus, prevention, partnerships, cultural respect, and empowerment—collectively shape the practice of nurses in this field. By adhering to these principles, CHNs can effectively contribute to the health and well-being of populations, ultimately leading to healthier communities.

Community Health Models

Community health models serve as frameworks for understanding and addressing the multifaceted health needs of populations within a community setting. These models emphasize the integration of various health determinants, including social, economic, and environmental factors, which collectively influence community health outcomes [6, 8]. By leveraging a holistic approach, community health models aim to foster collaborative efforts among healthcare providers, community leaders, and residents to improve health equity and access to care.

One fundamental aspect of community health models is their focus on prevention and early intervention. By identifying at-risk populations and implementing targeted interventions, these models strive to mitigate health disparities and enhance overall community well-being. This preventive approach often involves health education programs, vaccination campaigns, and screening initiatives designed to detect and address potential health issues before they escalate into more severe conditions.

A key component of community health models is the recognition of the social determinants of health, which include factors such as income, education, employment, and housing [1]. These determinants play a crucial role in shaping health behaviors and outcomes. Community health models advocate for policies and interventions that address these determinants, thereby promoting healthier lifestyles and reducing the burden of disease. For instance, initiatives aimed at improving access to nutritious food, safe housing, and quality education can have a profound impact on community health.

Moreover, community health models underscore the importance of cultural respect in healthcare delivery [5, 11]. By acknowledging and respecting the diverse cultural backgrounds of community members, healthcare providers can deliver more effective and personalized care. This culturally sensitive approach enhances patient engagement and trust, leading to better health outcomes and increased satisfaction with care.

Intersectoral collaboration is another cornerstone of community health models. By fostering partnerships among healthcare providers, government agencies, non-profit organizations, and community groups, these models facilitate the sharing of resources and expertise. Such collaborations enable the development and implementation of comprehensive health strategies that address the unique needs of each community.

Technology and data analytics also play a pivotal role in community health models [14, 15]. The use of electronic health records, geographic information systems, and health informatics allows for the collection and analysis of data to identify health trends, track the effectiveness of interventions, and allocate resources efficiently. This data-driven approach enhances decision-making and enables the continuous improvement of community health initiatives.

In addition, community health models advocate for the empowerment of individuals and communities to take charge of their health [5]. Through participatory approaches, community members are encouraged to engage in health planning and decision-making processes. This empowerment fosters a sense of ownership and responsibility, which is essential for the sustainability of health interventions.

Overall, community health models provide a comprehensive framework for addressing the complex health challenges faced by communities. By integrating prevention, cultural respect, intersectoral collaboration, and data-driven strategies, these models aim to improve health outcomes and promote health equity. As such, they represent a vital component of public health efforts to create healthier, more resilient communities.

Future Trends

In the rapidly evolving field of community health nursing, several emerging trends are shaping the future of practice and policy. These trends are driven by technological advancements, demographic shifts, and an increasing emphasis on preventive care and holistic health approaches [7, 10–14]. As the healthcare landscape continues to transform, CHNs are adapting to new roles and responsibilities that extend beyond traditional care delivery.

One significant trend is the integration of technology into community health practices. The proliferation of digital health tools, such as telehealth platforms, mobile health applications, and electronic health records, is revolutionizing how care is delivered and managed [7, 12, 14]. These technologies enable CHNs to reach underserved populations, facilitate remote monitoring of chronic conditions, and enhance patient engagement and education. As technology continues to advance, CHNs will increasingly leverage data analytics to identify health trends, tailor interventions, and improve health outcomes.

Demographic changes are also influencing the future of community health nursing [11]. The aging population presents unique challenges and opportunities for healthcare providers. As life expectancy increases, there is a growing need for services that address the complex health needs of older adults. CHNs are at the forefront of developing programs that promote healthy aging, manage chronic diseases, and support caregivers. Additionally, the increasing diversity of the population requires culturally competent care that respects and responds to the varied beliefs and practices of different communities.

The focus on preventive care and health promotion is another key trend shaping the future of community health nursing [10, 12]. There is a shift from reactive, illness-centered care to proactive, wellness-focused approaches. CHNs are playing a pivotal role in implementing strategies that encourage healthy lifestyles, reduce risk factors, and prevent the onset of diseases. This includes conducting community assessments, designing health education programs, and advocating for policies that address social determinants of health.

Interprofessional collaboration is becoming increasingly important in community health settings. As healthcare becomes more integrated, CHNs are working alongside other professionals, such as social workers, nutritionists, and mental health counselors, to provide comprehensive care. This collaborative approach enables the delivery of holistic care that addresses the physical, mental, and social aspects of health. By fostering partnerships with various stakeholders, CHNs are enhancing the quality and accessibility of care for individuals and communities.

Finally, environmental health is gaining attention as a critical component of community health nursing [3, 5]. The impact of climate change, pollution, and other environmental factors on health is prompting CHNs to advocate for sustainable practices and policies. Nurses are involved in educating communities about environmental risks, promoting eco-friendly behaviors, and participating in initiatives that aim to create healthier environments. Figure 1.2 summarizes the key emerging trends in community health nursing.

In conclusion, the future of community health nursing is characterized by innovation, collaboration, and a commitment to improving population health. As these trends continue to evolve, CHNs will play a vital role in shaping a healthcare system that is responsive to the needs of diverse populations and capable of addressing the challenges of the twenty-first century.

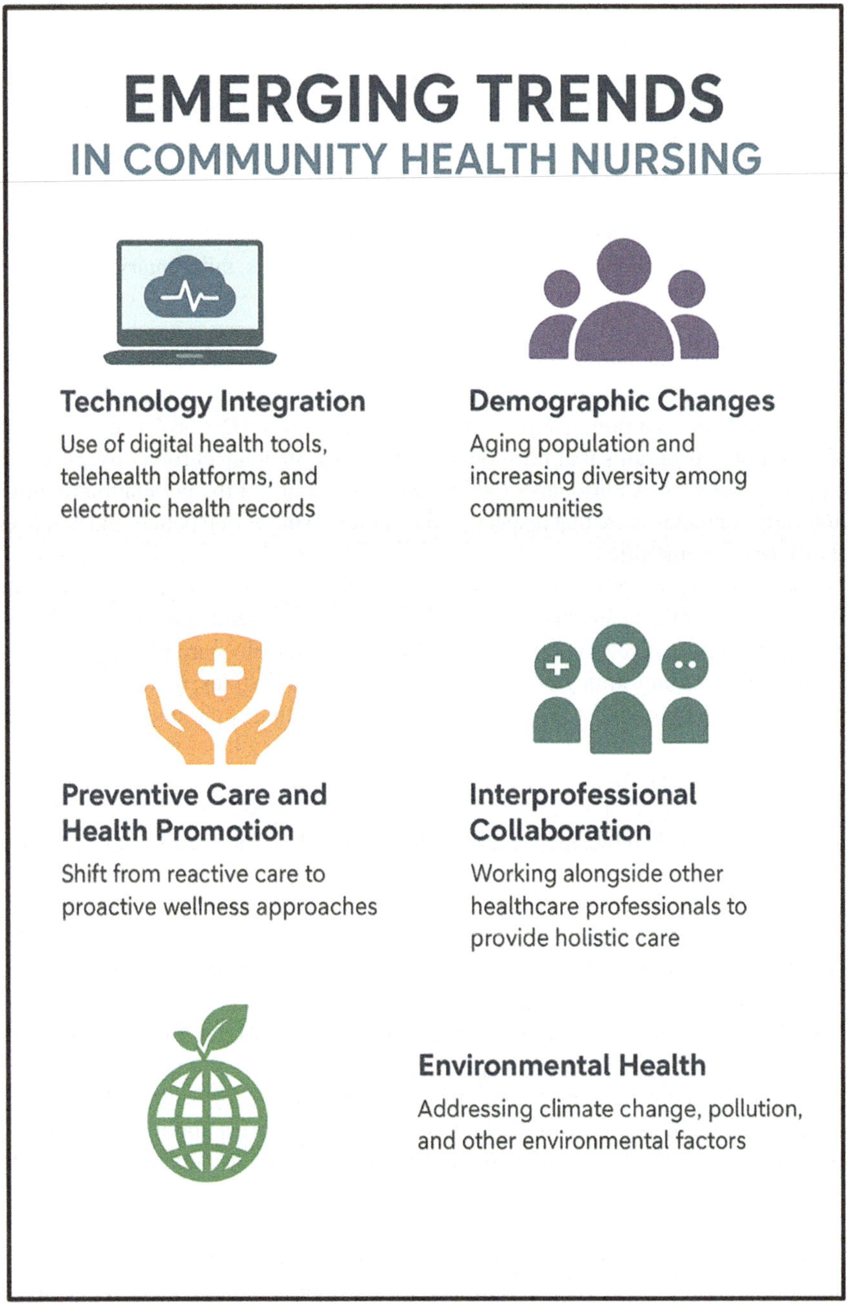

Fig. 1.2 Key emerging trends in community health nursing

References

1. Nies MA, McEwen M. Community/public health nursing: promoting the health of populations. 8th ed. St. Louis: Elsevier; 2023.
2. Stanhope M, Lancaster J. Public health nursing: population-centered health care in the community. 10th ed. St. Louis: Elsevier Health Sciences; 2019.
3. Stilwell B. Global health and nursing: a new narrative for the 21st century. 1st ed. St. Louis: Elsevier; 2025.
4. Aladani N. Assessment of nursing practice environment in primary healthcare centers in Saudi Arabia: a cross-sectional study. SAGE Open. 2023;9:1–9.
5. Allender J, Rector C, Warner K. Community & public health nursing: promoting the public's health. Philadelphia: Lippincott Williams & Wilkins; 2013.
6. Lundy K, Janes S. Community health nursing: caring for the public's health. 3rd ed. Burlington: Jones & Bartlett Learning; 2016.
7. Kulbok PA, Thatcher E, Park E, Meszaros P. Evolving public health nursing roles: focus on community participatory health promotion and prevention. Online J Issues Nurs. 2012;17(2):1. https://doi.org/10.3912/OJIN.Vol17No02Man01.
8. Maurer F, Smith C. Community/public health nursing practice: health for families and populations. 5th ed. St. Louis: Saunders; 2012.
9. World Health Organization. Nursing and midwifery [Internet]. Geneva: WHO; 2024. https://www.who.int/news-room/fact-sheets/detail/nursing-and-midwifery. Accessed 12 Feb 2026.
10. Almadani N. Assessment of nursing practice environment in primary healthcare centers in Saudi Arabia: a cross-sectional study. SAGE Open. 2023;13:1–9. https://doi.org/10.1177/21582440231208930.
11. Aljohani K. Community health nursing in Saudi Arabia: practices and learning needs. Risk Manag Healthc Policy. 2024;17:3239–3245. https://doi.org/10.2147/RMHP.S504277.
12. Hussain Y, Zubayd H, Zubay S, Alghamdi S, Alyami H, Al Rizq H, et al. Advancing primary healthcare in Saudi Arabia: integrating nursing, dental, and community health approaches in line with Vision 2030. Rev Contemp Philos. 2024;23(2):1254–1268.
13. Alsadaan N, Jones L, Kimpton A. Challenges facing the nursing profession in Saudi Arabia: an integrative review. Nurs Rep. 2021;11(2):395–403. https://doi.org/10.3390/nursrep11020038.
14. Alruwaili M, Ali R, Shahbal S, Alotaibi S, Althiyabi N, Aldosari M, et al. Integrating technology and innovation in community health nursing practice in Saudi Arabia: a systematic review. J Namib Stud Hist Polit Cult. 2023;35:2829–2852.
15. Elmorshedy H, AlAmrani H, Hassan M, Fayed A, Albrecht S. Contemporary public image of the nursing profession in Saudi Arabia. BMC Nurs. 2020;19:47. https://doi.org/10.1186/s12912-020-00442-w.

2 Cultural Respect in Community Health Nursing

Learning Objectives

By the end of this chapter, students will be able to:

1. Define and explain the concept of cultural diversity and its implications for health behaviors, healthcare access, and health equity in community health nursing.
2. Analyze how cultural beliefs, values, language, religion, and socioeconomic factors influence patients' perceptions of illness, health-seeking behaviors, and adherence to treatment within diverse populations.
3. Differentiate between the key components of cultural respect and apply these principles to the delivery of culturally responsive care.
4. Critically evaluate the role of cultural respect as an ethical and professional foundation in community health nursing, emphasizing its importance in reducing health disparities and improving patient outcomes.
5. Demonstrate effective communication strategies that incorporate cultural respect, active listening, use of interpreters, clear language, and appropriate nonverbal communication across diverse cultural contexts.
6. Design and implement culturally appropriate community engagement strategies that build trust, foster participation, and empower communities to identify and address their own health priorities.
7. Assess the impact of institutional and policy-level interventions on healthcare delivery and equity.
8. Interpret and discuss real-world case studies that illustrate the challenges and best practices in culturally competent community health nursing within rural, urban, and multicultural contexts.
9. Examine the cultural landscape of Middle Eastern and Saudi communities, including religion, family structure, gender norms, traditional medicine, and linguistic diversity, to enhance culturally sensitive nursing practice.

R. I. Ashgar, *Community Health Nursing: Principles, Practices, and Perspectives*,
https://doi.org/10.1007/978-3-032-30791-0_2

10. Evaluate how Saudi Arabia's Vision 2030 reforms and modernization efforts are reshaping cultural practices, healthcare delivery, and the role of community health nurses in promoting cultural respect, inclusion, and health equity.

Understanding Cultural Diversity

Cultural diversity is a critical aspect of community health nursing, influencing both the provision and reception of healthcare services. It encompasses a wide array of cultural differences that include, but are not limited to, ethnicity, language, religion, and socioeconomic status [1]. Understanding these differences is essential for healthcare professionals to deliver effective and equitable care. This requires a comprehensive approach that integrates cultural respect into all levels of healthcare delivery [2, 3]. Recognizing cultural diversity involves acknowledging the unique cultural characteristics and health beliefs that patients bring to the healthcare setting. These characteristics can significantly affect health behaviors and attitudes towards healthcare systems [4]. For instance, cultural beliefs can influence a patient's willingness to seek medical treatment, adherence to prescribed therapies, and perceptions of illness and wellness. Therefore, healthcare providers must develop cultural respect, which is the ability to understand, communicate with, and effectively interact with people across cultures [5].

The development of cultural respect begins with cultural awareness, which involves self-examination and in-depth exploration of one's own cultural and professional background [1, 6]. This process helps in identifying personal biases, prejudices, and assumptions about individuals who are different. Cultural knowledge, another component of cultural respect, involves seeking and obtaining a sound educational foundation concerning the various worldviews of different cultures [1, 6]. This knowledge can be obtained through direct interaction with patients from diverse backgrounds, as well as through formal education and training programs. Cultural skill is another essential component, referring to the ability to collect relevant cultural data regarding the patient's health issue and perform a culturally based physical assessment [7]. This requires healthcare providers to engage in culturally sensitive communication and employ culturally appropriate interventions. The use of interpreters, culturally relevant health education materials, and culturally tailored health promotion programs are examples of strategies to enhance cultural respect in healthcare settings.

In addition to individual efforts, healthcare institutions play a significant role in promoting cultural respect [8–10]. Institutions can implement policies and practices that support cultural diversity, such as recruiting a diverse workforce, providing ongoing cultural respect training, and fostering an inclusive environment where cultural differences are respected and valued.

Moreover, policy advocacy is crucial in addressing systemic barriers to healthcare access and equity for culturally diverse populations [11]. Evaluating the effectiveness of cultural respect interventions is vital to ensure that they meet the intended goals of improving healthcare outcomes and reducing health disparities [8, 12]. This involves continuous assessment and adaptation of strategies based on feedback from patients and healthcare providers. Research and evidence-based practices are essential in guiding these efforts and in understanding the complex relationship between cultural diversity and health outcomes. Ultimately, understanding cultural diversity is not a static goal but an ongoing process that requires commitment and dedication from healthcare professionals and organizations alike [4, 7, 9]. By fostering an environment of respect and inclusion, community health nursing can enhance the quality of care provided to all individuals, regardless of their cultural background. This commitment not only improves patient satisfaction and health outcomes but also strengthens the overall healthcare system by promoting equity and social justice.

Culturally Competent Care

The provision of culturally competent care represents a fundamental aspect of community health nursing, necessitating a nuanced understanding and integration of diverse cultural backgrounds into healthcare practices. This involves recognizing and respecting the unique cultural needs of individuals and communities, which can significantly influence health behaviors, health status, and the effectiveness of healthcare interventions. Culturally competent care is not merely an ethical obligation, but a critical component in achieving health equity and improving health outcomes for diverse populations [1].

Central to culturally competent care is the concept of cultural awareness, which requires healthcare providers to engage in self-reflection and recognize their own cultural biases and assumptions [13, 14]. This process enhances the ability to understand and appreciate the cultural perspectives of patients, thereby facilitating more effective communication and interaction. It involves acknowledging the cultural influences on health beliefs and practices, which can vary widely among different ethnic and cultural groups.

In addition to cultural awareness, cultural knowledge is essential for providing culturally competent care [4, 15–17]. This entails acquiring information about different cultural practices, health-related beliefs, and traditional healing practices. Healthcare providers must be knowledgeable about the cultural contexts of the communities they serve, which includes understanding the social, economic, and political factors that shape health behaviors and access to healthcare. This knowledge allows for the adaptation of healthcare practices to meet the specific needs of diverse populations.

Cultural skills are also vital in delivering culturally competent care [5, 18]. These skills enable healthcare providers to conduct culturally sensitive assessments and to communicate effectively with patients from diverse backgrounds. This includes using culturally appropriate language and communication techniques, as well as employing interpreters when necessary to ensure clear and accurate communication. Developing cultural skills enhances the ability to build trust and rapport with patients, which is crucial for effective healthcare delivery [19]. Furthermore, cultural encounters are a critical component of culturally competent care [7, 14]. These encounters provide healthcare providers with opportunities to engage directly with individuals from diverse cultural backgrounds, thereby gaining practical experience and insight. Through these interactions, providers can refine their cultural skills and knowledge, leading to more personalized and effective care. Cultural encounters also help to challenge stereotypes and reduce prejudices, fostering a more inclusive and respectful healthcare environment.

Finally, cultural desire is an intrinsic motivation that drives healthcare providers to become more culturally competent [14]. It reflects a genuine commitment to understanding and valuing cultural diversity, and a willingness to embrace cultural differences as an asset in healthcare delivery. Cultural desire encourages ongoing learning and adaptation, ensuring that healthcare practices remain relevant and responsive to the needs of diverse populations.

Incorporating culturally competent care into community health nursing requires a comprehensive approach that integrates cultural awareness, knowledge, skills, encounters, and desire. By doing so, healthcare providers can enhance their ability to deliver equitable and effective care, ultimately contributing to the overall health and well-being of the communities they serve. This approach not only improves patient satisfaction and health outcomes but also promotes social justice and health equity within the healthcare system. Figure 2.1 summarizes culturally competent care in community health nursing.

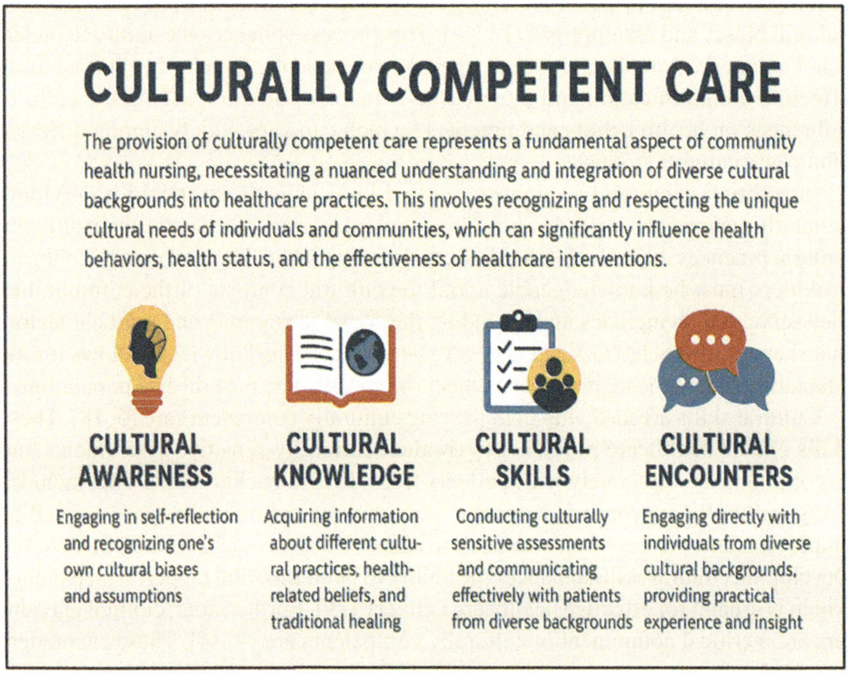

Fig. 2.1 Culturally competent care

Communication Strategies

Effective communication strategies are pivotal in community health nursing, facilitating the exchange of information between healthcare providers and the community [20]. These strategies are grounded in understanding the diverse cultural, social, and economic backgrounds of individuals within a community. By tailoring communication approaches, nurses can enhance engagement, promote health literacy, and ultimately improve health outcomes.

As demonstrated in Fig. 2.2, effective communication involves multiple strategies. Central to these strategies is the concept of cultural respect, which involves recognizing and respecting the cultural differences that influence how individuals perceive health and illness. Nurses must be adept at employing culturally appropriate communication techniques, including the use of language services such as translation and interpretation when necessary [20]. This ensures that all community members receive information in a manner that is both understandable and respectful of their cultural contexts.

Active listening is another fundamental component of effective communication in community health nursing [11]. By attentively listening to the concerns and needs of community members, nurses can gain valuable insights into the factors affecting their health. This approach not only builds trust but also enables nurses to tailor health messages to address specific issues pertinent to the community.

Moreover, the use of clear and simple language is essential in health communication [21]. Avoiding medical jargon and using terms that are easily understood by the general public can significantly enhance comprehension. Visual aids, such as diagrams and charts, can also be utilized to convey complex information more effectively, particularly in communities with low literacy levels.

The integration of technology in communication strategies has become increasingly important [20]. Digital platforms, including social media, mobile applications, and telehealth services, offer innovative ways to reach a broader audience. These tools can facilitate timely dissemination of health information, provide platforms for community engagement, and support remote consultations, thereby increasing accessibility to healthcare services.

Building strong community partnerships is another effective strategy. Collaborating with local organizations, schools, and religious institutions can help nurses reach diverse population segments and foster a sense of community ownership over health initiatives. These partnerships can also serve as channels for feedback, allowing nurses to continuously refine their communication strategies to better meet the needs of the community.

Health education is a critical aspect of communication strategies in community health nursing [22, 23]. By conducting workshops, seminars, and health fairs, nurses can educate community members about preventive measures, healthy lifestyle choices, and available health services. These educational efforts should be interactive and participatory, encouraging community members to ask questions and engage in discussions.

Feedback mechanisms are crucial for evaluating the effectiveness of communication strategies [24]. By soliciting feedback from community members, nurses can assess the

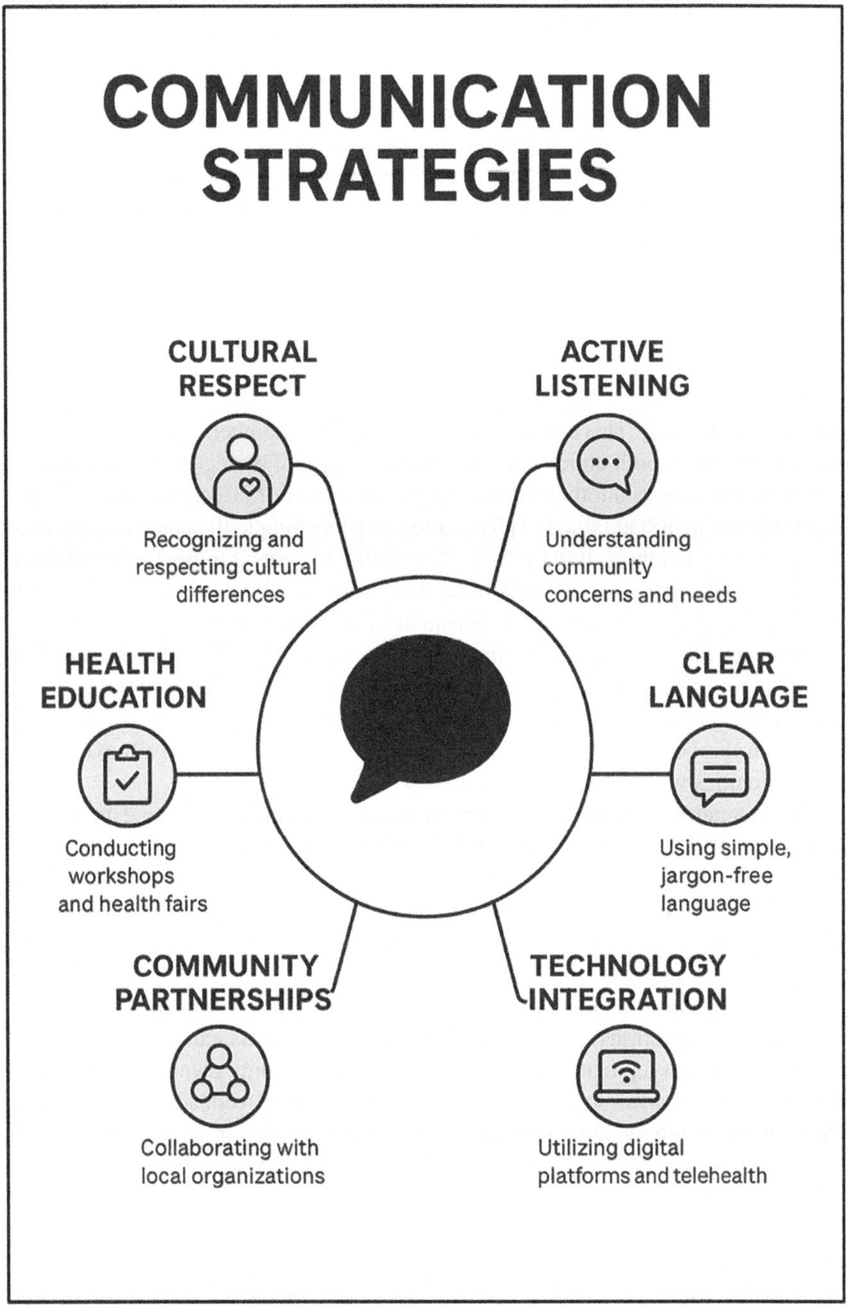

Fig. 2.2 Communication strategies

clarity and impact of their messages. This feedback can inform future communication efforts, ensuring they are more aligned with the community's preferences and needs.

In conclusion, effective communication strategies in community health nursing require a multifaceted approach that considers cultural respect, active listening, clear language, technology integration, community partnerships, and continuous feedback. By adopting these strategies, nurses can enhance their ability to communicate effectively with diverse communities, ultimately leading to improved health outcomes and stronger community relations.

Community Engagement

Community engagement is a critical component of community health nursing, serving as a bridge between healthcare providers and the populations they serve [25]. This engagement is characterized by proactive interactions with community members, fostering relationships that enhance mutual understanding and cooperation. It involves identifying community needs, priorities, and resources, thereby facilitating the development of tailored health interventions that are culturally sensitive and relevant.

A fundamental aspect of community engagement is the establishment of trust and rapport with community members. Trust is built through consistent, transparent, and respectful communication, which encourages community members to participate actively in health-related initiatives.

Engaging community leaders and stakeholders is particularly effective, as they can act as liaisons between the healthcare team and the broader community, advocating for health needs and mobilizing resources. Community health nurses (CHNs) employ various strategies to engage with communities effectively. One such strategy is participatory action research, which involves community members in all stages of the research process, from identifying issues to implementing solutions. This collaborative approach not only empowers communities but also ensures that health interventions are grounded in the lived experiences of the people they aim to serve [26]. Another critical strategy is the use of culturally competent care practices. CHNs must be aware of and sensitive to the cultural beliefs and practices of the communities they serve. This cultural respect enables nurses to design and implement health interventions that are more likely to be accepted and sustained by the community, as they respect and incorporate local traditions and values.

Moreover, community engagement in health extends to the development of community partnerships. These partnerships can be with other healthcare providers, local government agencies, educational institutions, and nongovernmental organizations. Such collaborations enhance the capacity of community health initiatives, allowing for a more comprehensive and coordinated approach to addressing health issues.

Evaluation and feedback are integral to community engagement efforts. Regular assessment of health interventions helps identify areas for improvement and ensures that the initiatives remain relevant to the community's evolving needs. Feedback from community members provides valuable insights into the effectiveness of health programs and can guide future engagement strategies.

In summary, community engagement in community health nursing is a dynamic and ongoing process that requires commitment, flexibility, and cultural sensitivity. By fostering strong relationships with community members and stakeholders, CHNs can facilitate meaningful health improvements, promote health equity, and empower communities to take charge of their health outcomes.

Case Studies

In the realm of community health nursing, case studies serve as an essential tool for understanding the multifaceted challenges and solutions encountered in real-world settings. These case studies illuminate the complex interplay of social, economic, and environmental factors that influence health outcomes within communities. Through detailed examination, they provide invaluable insights into the application of theoretical knowledge to practical scenarios, enhancing the competency and preparedness of CHNs.

One notable case involves the implementation of a community-based intervention aimed at reducing the prevalence of Type 2 diabetes in a rural population. The initiative, spearheaded by a team of CHNs, involved a comprehensive program that included nutritional education, physical activity promotion, and regular health screenings. The nurses worked collaboratively with local leaders to tailor the intervention to the community's cultural and economic context, ensuring greater acceptance and participation. The outcome was a significant reduction in new diabetes cases and improved management of existing conditions, demonstrating the efficacy of culturally sensitive, community-driven health interventions.

Another case study highlights the challenges faced by CHNs in urban settings, where high population density and socioeconomic disparities exacerbate health issues. In this scenario, nurses addressed the rising rates of asthma among children in a low-income neighborhood. By conducting home visits, they identified environmental triggers such as poor housing conditions and air pollution. The intervention involved educating families on asthma management, advocating for improved housing policies, and collaborating with local government to mitigate pollution sources. This multifaceted approach not only reduced asthma incidence but also empowered the community to advocate for healthier living conditions.

A third case study focuses on the role of CHNs in disaster response. Following a devastating hurricane, nurses were at the forefront of emergency response efforts in a coastal community. They provided immediate medical care, coordinated with relief organizations, and offered psychological support to affected individuals. The nurses' ability to rapidly assess community needs and mobilize resources was critical in mitigating the disaster's impact. This case underscores the importance of disaster preparedness training for CHNs, enabling them to effectively manage public health crises.

These case studies collectively highlight the diverse roles of CHNs in promoting health equity and resilience. They demonstrate the importance of community engagement, interdisciplinary collaboration, and adaptability in addressing public health challenges. By analyzing these scenarios, CHNs can refine their skills and strategies, ultimately contributing to healthier and more resilient communities.

Cultural Landscape of Middle Eastern Communities

Understanding the cultural landscape of Middle Eastern communities is fundamental to effective community health nursing. The region's diverse societies—spanning the Arabian Peninsula, Levant, and North Africa—share deep historical, religious, and linguistic ties, yet display remarkable variations in traditions, family structures, and healthcare practices [27]. For nurses and healthcare providers, cultural awareness forms the basis for respectful, patient-centered care that aligns with community norms and values.

The Cultural Foundation: Religion and Spirituality

Religion plays a central role in shaping the worldview of Middle Eastern populations. Islam is the predominant faith across the region, guiding daily life, social relations, and health behaviors. The Qur'an and Hadith provide moral frameworks that influence:

- Perceptions of illness as a test from God or a path to spiritual purification.
- Practices of hygiene and dietary restrictions (e.g., halal food, prohibition of alcohol).
- End-of-life care rituals and spiritual readiness for death.
- Use of prophetic or traditional medicine, such as honey, black seed, and cupping (Hijama).

Healthcare professionals must recognize the spiritual dimensions of care, ensuring that religious beliefs are respected and integrated into nursing practice. Additionally, some Middle Eastern countries include Christian, Druze, or other minority populations, requiring an inclusive approach that honors diverse faith traditions.

Family and Social Structures

Family remains the cornerstone of Middle Eastern society. Extended family networks often influence decision-making, caregiving, and social support systems [27]. Elders command respect, and collective decision-making is common, especially in health-related matters.

- Male guardianship traditions may influence women's health decisions in more conservative areas.
- Families frequently accompany patients during hospital stays, reflecting strong kinship bonds.

Nurses must navigate these dynamics with cultural sensitivity during communication, discharge planning, and home care.

Gender Norms and Modesty

Cultural expectations around gender and modesty shape healthcare interactions across the region.

- Female patients often prefer care from female nurses, especially in maternal or reproductive health.
- Physical examinations by opposite-gender staff typically require consent and sensitivity.
- Female nurses must balance professional duties with cultural norms that may limit cross-gender interaction.

Respect for modesty—through appropriate draping, privacy measures, and consent—is critical for maintaining patient trust and comfort.

Language and Communication

Arabic is the predominant language of the Middle East, but local dialects and minority languages (e.g., Kurdish, Persian, Berber) contribute to linguistic diversity.

- Effective communication requires awareness of verbal and nonverbal nuances, such as indirectness or limited eye contact between genders.
- In multicultural healthcare environments, interpreters and visual aids can improve understanding and patient engagement.

Urban–Rural and Socioeconomic Differences

The Middle East exhibits clear contrasts between urban and rural communities.

- Urban areas tend to adopt modern healthcare technologies and international health practices.
- Rural and nomadic communities may maintain traditional healing methods, have lower health literacy, and face access barriers.

Community health nurses (CHNs) must adapt their approaches to match local resources, education levels, and cultural expectations.

Traditional and Prophetic Medicine

Traditional healing remains integral to Middle Eastern culture. Practices such as Hijama (cupping), Ruqyah (spiritual healing), and herbal medicine coexist with modern medicine.

Nurses should acknowledge the cultural significance of these practices while ensuring patient safety, offering respectful guidance on potential interactions with prescribed treatments.

Saudi Arabia: A Distinct Cultural Context

Saudi Arabia exemplifies how Middle Eastern traditions intertwine with rapid modernization. The Kingdom's cultural identity is deeply rooted in Islam, tribal heritage, and evolving social dynamics shaped by Vision 2030 reforms [8]. For nurses working in Saudi communities, understanding this cultural context is essential to delivering respectful, effective, and patient-centered care.

Islamic Faith as the Cultural Foundation

Islam is not only the official religion but also the cornerstone of Saudi identity, law, and daily life. It influences perceptions of health, illness, death, and healing. The Qur'an and Hadith (sayings of Prophet Muhammad, peace be upon him) serve as moral and practical guides for many Saudis, shaping:

- Health beliefs (e.g., illness may be seen as a test from Allah or a means of purification).
- End-of-life care (e.g., belief in divine will and the importance of reciting prayers before death).
- Hygiene and cleanliness (e.g., ablution before prayer).
- Dietary habits (e.g., prohibition of pork and alcohol; preference for halal food).
- Use of alternative and prophetic medicine (e.g., honey, black seed, cupping [Hijama]).

Healthcare providers must understand and accommodate these beliefs to gain the trust of patients and families and avoid unintentional offense.

Tribal and Family Structures

Saudi society historically developed through tribal affiliations, and many social relationships are still shaped by extended family networks. Families often take collective responsibility for decision-making, especially concerning health matters.

- Male guardianship traditions may influence how decisions are made for female patients.
- Elders and patriarchs are respected and may be central figures in healthcare decisions.

- Families may accompany patients during hospital stays and play a strong advocacy role.

Understanding the importance of family dynamics is crucial for nurses during communication, discharge planning, and home care services.

Gender Norms and Modesty

Cultural and religious norms place a high value on modesty, particularly in interactions between men and women.

- Female patients may prefer care from female nurses, especially in areas such as maternal health, gynecology, or home visits.
- Physical examinations by opposite-gender staff are often avoided unless medically necessary, and consent is typically required.
- Female nurses must also navigate gender expectations when providing care to male patients, especially in more conservative regions.

Nurses should maintain sensitivity to these norms by seeking consent, using modest draping techniques, and involving same-gender staff whenever possible.

Language Diversity and Communication

Arabic is the official language, and most Saudi patients are Arabic speakers. However, healthcare settings often include staff and patients from a wide range of linguistic backgrounds due to a multicultural workforce.

- Nurses may encounter language barriers with patients from minority groups or migrant communities.
- Use of professional interpreters, visual aids, or Arabic language training for non-Arabic speaking nurses can significantly improve communication.
- For Saudi patients, effective communication also includes understanding nonverbal cues, which can differ from Western norms (e.g., indirectness, avoidance of eye contact with the opposite gender).

Urban–Rural Differences

Saudi Arabia exhibits cultural variations between urban centers such as Riyadh, Jeddah, and Dammam, and rural or remote regions such as Asir, Najran, or Northern Borders.

- Urban populations tend to be more exposed to global cultures and healthcare practices.

- Rural communities may retain more traditional healing practices, have stronger tribal affiliations, and face limited access to healthcare services.

CHNs must tailor their approach to match the literacy levels, beliefs, and resources available in each locality.

Cultural Diversity Within the Kingdom

In addition to Saudis, the Kingdom is home to millions of expatriates from countries such as the Philippines, India, Pakistan, Bangladesh, Egypt, Sudan, and Indonesia. This diversity extends to patients and healthcare workers alike.

- Nurses may care for patients with varied religious backgrounds (e.g., Christians, Hindus, Buddhists) and practices.
- Cultural sensitivity must also apply to non-Saudi patient populations, ensuring equitable and inclusive care regardless of nationality or faith.

Role of Traditional and Prophetic Medicine

Many Saudis continue to rely on prophetic medicine, often alongside conventional medical treatments. Practices such as:

- Hijama (cupping)
- Ruqyah (spiritual healing using Qur'anic verses)
- Herbal remedies and diet-based healing

While these are often faith-based and meaningful to patients, nurses should address them respectfully, assess for potential interactions with prescribed treatments, and offer education without dismissing cultural beliefs.

Influence of Vision 2030 and Health Modernization

Saudi Arabia's Vision 2030 initiative is reshaping the healthcare system by promoting preventive care, digital health, and workforce development. With more women joining the workforce, increasing health awareness campaigns, and expanding public health initiatives, cultural expectations are also evolving.

- Nurses are increasingly expected to be community educators and advocates, not just caregivers.
- Cultural respect now includes being attuned to generational shifts, digital health literacy, and urbanization impacts on health behaviors.

Regional and Cultural Diversity Within Saudi Arabia

Saudi Arabia is a vast and diverse nation whose cultural identity is shaped by geography, history, tribal heritage, and rapid modernization. While united by a shared Islamic faith and Arabic language, the Kingdom's regions exhibit distinct traditions, dialects, cuisines, dress styles, and social practices that influence community life and health behaviors [28]. Understanding these regional variations is essential for community health nurses (CHNs), educators, and policymakers seeking to deliver culturally competent care across the country's varied settings.

Geographic Overview

Saudi Arabia spans over two million square kilometers, encompassing deserts, mountains, coastal plains, oases, and islands. Its five primary regions—Central (Najd), Western (Hijaz), Eastern (Ash Sharqiyah), Southern (Asir, Jazan, Najran, and Al-Baha), and Northern (Al-Jawf, Tabuk, Hail, and Northern Borders)—each developed unique cultural identities influenced by geography, trade routes, tribal affiliations, and exposure to external cultures (see Fig. 2.3). Historically, these regions

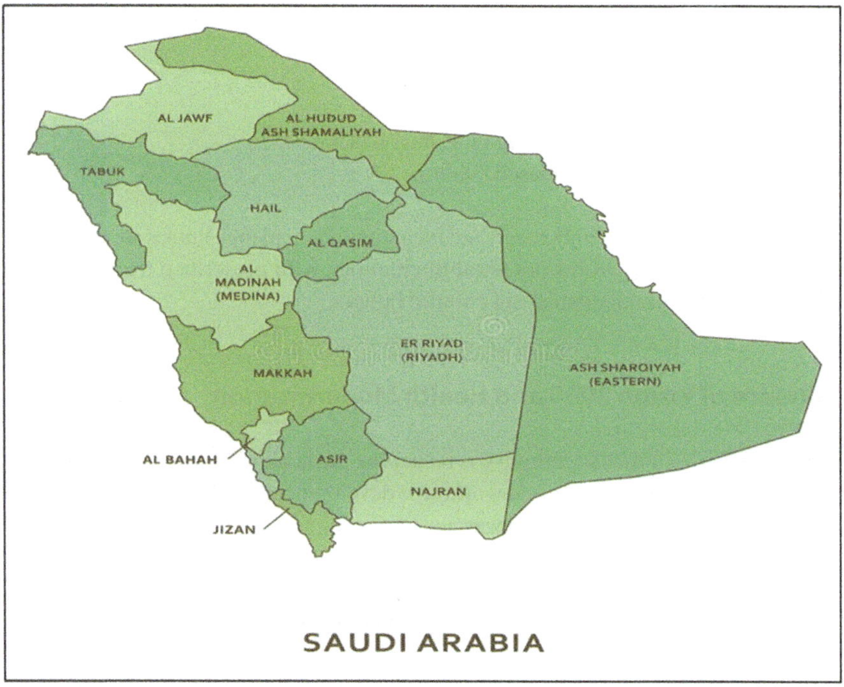

Fig. 2.3 Regions of Saudi Arabia

developed semi-independently, and elements of their distinct identities remain evident in contemporary Saudi society [28].

Central Region (Najd): The political and cultural heart of the Kingdom, home to the capital Riyadh. Characterized by a conservative interpretation of Islam and a strong tribal legacy, Najd emphasizes traditional values, hospitality, and kinship.

Western Region (Hijaz): Encompasses Makkah, Madinah, and Jeddah—the spiritual and historical center of Islam. The region's long history of pilgrimage and trade has created a cosmopolitan culture influenced by pilgrims and merchants from Africa, Asia, and the Mediterranean.

Eastern Region (Ash Sharqiyah): Known for its oil wealth, industrial cities, and coastal culture along the Arabian Gulf. It has a tradition of openness due to maritime trade.

Southern Regions (Asir, Jazan, Najran, and Al-Baha): Distinguished by mountainous terrain, terraced agriculture, and strong tribal identities. The region is characterized by its colorful attire and distinctive architecture.

Northern Regions (Al-Jawf, Tabuk, Hail, and Northern Borders): Known for its Bedouin heritage, archaeological sites, and cooler climate. Northern tribes have preserved nomadic traditions and hospitality as core cultural values.

Cultural Expressions and Social Practices

Language and Dialects: Although the Arabic language serves as a unifying element across Saudi Arabia, significant regional linguistic variations reflect the country's cultural diversity and historical development. The major dialect groups—Najdi, Hijazi, Gulf (Eastern), and Southern Arabic—are closely tied to regional identity, social interaction, and heritage. These dialects not only convey local distinctiveness but also influence communication dynamics within healthcare settings, where effective provider–patient interaction depends heavily on linguistic understanding and cultural sensitivity.

Najdi Arabic, spoken predominantly in the central region, is often perceived as the most conservative and linguistically "pure" form of Saudi Arabic. It tends to preserve traditional expressions, formal structures, and pronunciations rooted in classical Arabic [29]. Speakers of Najdi Arabic may also exhibit a communication style that values formality and respect for hierarchy, which can affect clinical encounters and patient engagement.

Hijazi Arabic, spoken in the western region—including Makkah, Madinah, and Jeddah—displays greater linguistic diversity. Owing to the region's historical exposure to international pilgrims and merchants, the Hijazi dialect incorporates numerous loanwords from languages such as Turkish, Persian, Urdu, and English. This linguistic openness mirrors the cosmopolitan nature of the Hijaz and often corresponds with more expressive and interactive communication patterns in healthcare contexts [30].

Gulf Arabic (Eastern dialect), prevalent in Ash Sharqiyah, reflects long-standing maritime and trade connections with the broader Arabian Gulf. It contains lexical similarities with dialects from Kuwait, Bahrain, and Qatar, and its speakers may demonstrate pragmatic communication styles shaped by cross-cultural exchanges.

Southern dialects, including those spoken in Asir, Jazan, Najran, and Al-Baha, display the greatest phonological and lexical variation within the Kingdom. Influenced by the region's mountainous geography and tribal history, these dialects may differ considerably from Standard Arabic, occasionally presenting comprehension challenges for nonlocal speakers.

From a healthcare perspective, awareness of these linguistic distinctions is vital. Community health nurses (CHNs) and other professionals must not only understand regional vocabulary differences but also appreciate the cultural meanings embedded in speech patterns, tone, and modes of address. Linguistic competence thus forms a key component of culturally responsive care, supporting trust-building, accurate health education, and patient adherence to treatment plans.

Dress and Attire: While the formal national attire in Saudi Arabia consists of the thobe for men and the abaya for women, traditional clothing styles vary subtly across the country's regions. In the Hijaz, lighter fabrics are preferred, reflecting the coastal climate and cosmopolitan influences. The Central Region (Najd) favors simple, elegant designs in neutral tones that reflect Bedouin traditions and desert practicality. In the Eastern Province (Ash Sharqiyah), attire often incorporates Gulf-style elements, such as the decorative embroidery influenced by maritime trade and contact with neighboring Gulf cultures. The Southern regions—including Asir, Jazan, Najran, and Al-Baha—are known for their vibrant textiles, colorful dresses, and ornate silver jewelry that reveal strong Yemeni and tribal influences. In the Northern regions—Al-Jawf, Tabuk, Hail, and the Northern Borders—traditional garments are often made from heavier fabrics suited to cooler desert nights, with distinct embroidery patterns that convey tribal identity. These regional variations are more than aesthetic; they embody local heritage, climate adaptation, and enduring expressions of social belonging and cultural pride.

Cuisine and Hospitality: Food occupies a central place in Saudi Arabian social and cultural life, functioning not only as a means of sustenance but also as a powerful expression of identity, heritage, and communal values. Traditional cuisine reflects the Kingdom's regional diversity, with dishes and culinary practices shaped by geography, climate, and historical patterns of trade and migration. While kabsa—a spiced rice dish typically prepared with meat or chicken—has achieved the status of a national staple, each region retains distinctive culinary traditions that continue to symbolize local identity and pride.

In the Central Region (Najd)—the political and cultural heartland of Saudi Arabia—cuisine and hospitality practices reflect the region's desert environment, tribal heritage, and long-standing emphasis on simplicity and generosity. Traditional Najdi cuisine developed around the availability of locally sourced ingredients such as wheat, dates, dairy, and lamb, leading to the creation of hearty, nutritionally dense dishes designed to sustain people through harsh climatic conditions. Among the most prominent dishes are jareesh (cracked wheat cooked with meat or chicken), margoog (a stew of meat and vegetables thickened with whole-wheat dough), and hanini (a date-and-butter dessert traditionally consumed in winter). These foods exemplify both resourcefulness and a deep connection to agrarian life.

In the Hijaz, dishes such as mandi (slow-cooked spiced meat with rice) and saleeg (a creamy rice and milk-based dish similar to risotto) are particularly prominent. The Hijazi palate has been influenced by centuries of contact with pilgrims and merchants from Africa, Asia, and the Mediterranean, resulting in a cuisine characterized by rich flavors and diverse ingredients.

The Eastern Region (Ash Sharqiyah), situated along the Arabian Gulf, is known for its abundant seafood dishes, a culinary legacy of the region's maritime traditions. Dates and date-based products also hold special cultural and economic significance, reflecting both the region's agricultural heritage and its role in local hospitality practices.

In the Southern regions—including Asir, Jazan, Najran, and Al-Baha—distinctive mountain and agricultural environments have given rise to hearty, traditional foods such as areekah (a wheat and honey-based dish) and aseedah (a dense porridge made from wheat or sorghum). These dishes are often associated with communal gatherings and seasonal celebrations, reinforcing social cohesion and intergenerational continuity.

Across all regions, hospitality remains a defining cultural value. The act of welcoming guests with Arabic coffee (gahwa) and dates symbolizes generosity, respect, and social solidarity. Coffee serving is often accompanied by specific rituals—such as the order of pouring, the number of cups offered, and the use of ornate dallah (coffee pots)—which carry cultural meanings associated with honor and mutual respect. In both domestic and public contexts, these customs reflect broader social ethics emphasizing warmth, reciprocity, and the moral importance of caring for guests.

In the context of community health and social well-being, understanding such culinary and hospitality traditions enables health professionals to approach nutrition education, dietary interventions, and patient engagement in ways that respect and integrate local cultural values.

Urban–Rural Health Differences

Health outcomes and healthcare access in Saudi Arabia vary significantly between urban and rural populations, reflecting disparities in infrastructure, service availability, socioeconomic conditions, and health literacy. The Kingdom's rapid urbanization—driven by economic diversification and modernization—has concentrated healthcare resources and professionals in major cities such as Riyadh, Jeddah, and Dammam, while rural and remote areas continue to face challenges related to workforce shortages, limited health facilities, and reduced accessibility to specialized services [31].

Urban residents generally benefit from higher-quality healthcare infrastructure, greater access to tertiary hospitals, and a wider range of preventive and specialty services. These populations also tend to have higher educational attainment, income levels, and health awareness, which contribute to improved health-seeking behaviors and better management of chronic conditions such as diabetes and hypertension. However, urbanization has also been associated with the growing prevalence of non-communicable diseases (NCDs), obesity, and sedentary lifestyles, particularly among younger adults and women [32].

In contrast, rural communities—particularly those in the southern, northern, and peripheral regions—experience higher burdens of maternal and child health challenges, delayed disease detection, and limited access to emergency or specialized care [32]. Transportation barriers and shortages of healthcare personnel further exacerbate inequities in rural service delivery. Traditional beliefs, linguistic diversity, and varying levels of health literacy can also influence rural health behaviors and perceptions of medical care, underscoring the importance of culturally sensitive community health interventions.

Recent national initiatives, including Saudi Vision 2030 and the Health Sector Transformation Program, have prioritized addressing these disparities by decentralizing health services, investing in telemedicine, and expanding primary healthcare centers in underserved areas. These reforms aim to improve equity in health outcomes and ensure that rural populations receive care aligned with national quality and accessibility standards [33].

From a CHN perspective, understanding the social, cultural, and infrastructural determinants underlying urban–rural health differences is essential for promoting equitable care. CHNs play a pivotal role in outreach, health education, and disease prevention programs that bridge these gaps—particularly through community engagement, culturally tailored health promotion, and collaboration with local leaders to enhance trust and participation in preventive health initiatives.

Cultural Evolution Under Vision 2030

Saudi Arabia's Vision 2030 initiative has accelerated social transformation and health modernization. The program emphasizes preventive care, public health promotion, and diversification of the healthcare workforce.

- Health campaigns now address chronic diseases such as diabetes, obesity, and hypertension.
- Public health education integrates digital tools and community engagement.
- Cultural respect is increasingly recognized as a core skill in nursing curricula and healthcare training.

While modernization is reshaping daily life, cultural continuity remains strong—traditions of faith, hospitality, and family cohesion endure across all regions.

Implications for Community Health Nursing

Recognizing regional and cultural diversity within Saudi Arabia enables nurses to deliver equitable, context-sensitive care. Key implications include:

- Cultural Adaptation: Tailoring health messages to reflect local dialects, beliefs, and practices.
- Community Engagement: Collaborating with tribal leaders, elders, and family networks to support public health initiatives.

- Gender Sensitivity: Ensuring comfort, privacy, and consent in gendered interactions.
- Holistic Practice: Respecting traditional healing while promoting evidence-based practice.

Culturally competent community health nursing not only improves health outcomes but also strengthens trust between healthcare providers and Saudi communities.

References

1. Leininger M. Transcultural nursing: concepts, theories, research and practice. New York: McGraw-Hill Medical; 2002.
2. Aldhafeeri YG, Aldhafeeri JS, Alenazi MF, Alzabni KA, Aldhafeeri A, Alanazi S, Al-Ruwaili F. Culturally informed mental healthcare: Saudi nursing embracing Vision 2030's diversity goals. Rev Contemp Philos. 2024;23(2):844–57.
3. Almutairi AF, Rodney P. Critical cultural competence for culturally diverse workforces: toward equitable and peaceful health care. ANS Adv Nurs Sci. 2013;36(3):200–12. https://doi.org/10.1097/ANS.0b013e31829edd51.
4. Chae D, Kim J, Kim S, Lee J, Park S. Effectiveness of cultural competence educational interventions on health professionals and patient outcomes: a systematic review. Jpn J Nurs Sci. 2020;17(3):e12326 https://doi.org/10.1111/jjns.12326.
5. Osmancevic S, Steiner LM, Großschädl F, Lohrmann C, Schoberer D. The effectiveness of cultural competence interventions in nursing: a systematic review and meta-analysis. Int J Nurs Stud. 2025;167:105079 https://doi.org/10.1016/j.ijnurstu.2025.105079.
6. Campinha-Bacote J. The process of cultural competence in the delivery of healthcare services: a model of care. J Transcult Nurs. 2002;13(3):181–201. https://doi.org/10.1177/10459602013003003.
7. Engebretson J, Mahoney J, Carlson ED. Cultural competence in the era of evidence-based practice. J Prof Nurs. 2008;24(3):172–78. https://doi.org/10.1016/j.profnurs.2007.10.012.
8. Albougami AS, Alotaibi JS. Review of culture issues and challenges affecting nursing practice in Saudi Arabia. Malays J Nurs. 2020;11(4):47–56. https://doi.org/10.31674/mjn.2020.v11i04.009.
9. Falatah R, Al-Harbi L, Alhalal E. The association between cultural competency, structural empowerment, and effective communication among nurses in Saudi Arabia: a cross-sectional correlational study. Nurs Rep. 2022;12(2):281–90. https://doi.org/10.3390/nursrep12020028.
10. Gradellini C, Gómez-Cantarino S, Domínguez-Isabel P, Molina-Gallego B, Mecugni D, Ugarte-Gurrutxaga MI. Cultural competence and cultural sensitivity education in university nursing courses: a scoping review. Front Psychol. 2021;12:682920 https://doi.org/10.3389/fpsyg.2021.682920.
11. Alshammari M, Duff J, Guilhermino M. Barriers to nurse–patient communication in Saudi Arabia: an integrative review. BMC Nurs. 2019;18:61. https://doi.org/10.1186/s12912-019-0385-4.
12. Clarke PN, McFarland MR, Andrews MM, Leininger M. Caring: reflections on the impact of the culture care theory by McFarland & Andrews and a conversation with Leininger. Nurs Sci Q. 2009;22(3):233–9. https://doi.org/10.1177/0894318409337020.
13. Kaihlanen AM, Hietapakka L, Heponiemi T. Increasing cultural awareness: nurses' perceptions of cultural competence training. BMC Nurs. 2019;18:38. https://doi.org/10.1186/s12912-019-0363-x.
14. Sharifi N, Adib-Hajbaghery M, Najafi M. Cultural competence in nursing: a concept analysis. Int J Nurs Stud. 2019;99:103386 https://doi.org/10.1016/j.ijnurstu.2019.103386.
15. Cruz JP, Alquwez N, Cruz CP, Felicilda-Reynaldo RFD, Vitorino LM, Islam SMS. Cultural competence among nursing students in Saudi Arabia: a cross-sectional study. Int Nurs Rev. 2017;64:215–23. https://doi.org/10.1111/inr.12370.

16. Horvat L, Horey D, Romios P, Kis-Rigo J. Cultural competence education for health professionals. Cochrane Database Syst Rev. 2014;5:CD009405 https://doi.org/10.1002/14651858.CD009405.pub2.
17. Ličen S, Prosen M. The development of cultural competences in nursing students and their significance in shaping the future work environment: a pilot study. BMC Med Educ. 2023;23:819. https://doi.org/10.1186/s12909-023-04800-5.
18. Zeleke T, Wudu M, Bekalu Y, Wondifraw EB, Bazie G. Cultural competence and associated factors among nurses in public hospitals of South Wollo zone, Northeast Ethiopia: a multicenter cross-sectional study. BMC Nurs. 2024;23:487. https://doi.org/10.1186/s12912-024-02162-x.
19. Halabi J, Nilsson J, Lepp M. Professional competence among registered nurses working in hospitals in Saudi Arabia and their experiences of quality of nursing care and patient safety. J Transcult Nurs. 2021;32(4):425–33. https://doi.org/10.1177/1043659621992845.
20. Theron L, Shopo KD, Ngami O. Exploring perceptions of communication among culturally diverse nurses in Saudi Arabia. J Transcult Nurs. 2025;36(2):121–33. https://doi.org/10.1177/10436596241291839.
21. Shen Z. Cultural competence models and cultural competence assessment instruments in nursing: a literature review. J Transcult Nurs. 2015;26(3):308–21. https://doi.org/10.1177/1043659614524790.
22. Kim Y, Lee H. The effectiveness of a cultural competence training program for public health nurses using intervention mapping. J Korean Acad Community Health Nurs. 2016;27(4):410–22. https://doi.org/10.12799/jkachn.2016.27.4.410.
23. Purnell L. The Purnell model for cultural competence. J Transcult Nurs. 2002;13(3):193–201. https://doi.org/10.1177/10459602013003006.
24. Higginbottom GM, Richter MS, Mogale RS, Ortiz L, Young S, Mollel O. Identification of nursing assessment models/tools validated in clinical practice for use with diverse ethno-cultural groups: an integrative review. BMC Nurs. 2011;10:16. https://doi.org/10.1186/1472-6955-10-16.
25. Nies MA, McEwen M. Community/public health nursing: promoting the health of populations. 8th ed. St. Louis: Elsevier; 2023.
26. Ashgar R. Community-based participatory research in cardiovascular disease prevention for middle-aged women: a systematic review. Heart Int. 2025;19(1):12–9. https://doi.org/10.17925/HI.2025.19.1.1.
27. Pappé I. The modern Middle East: a social and cultural history. 3rd ed. London: Routledge; 2014. https://doi.org/10.4324/9781315858340
28. Alsulami ND. Factors contributing to some cultural dimensions of Saudi Arabia. Am Int J Contemp Res. 2019;9(4):32–8. https://doi.org/10.30845/AIJCR.V9N4P4.
29. Al-Rojaie Y. Perceptual mapping of linguistic variation in Saudi Arabic dialects. Pozn Stud Contemp Linguist. 2021;57(4):471–517. https://doi.org/10.1515/psicl-2021-0019.
30. Alahmadi SD. Loanwords in the urban Meccan Hijazi dialect: lexical variation by sex, age, and education. Int J Engl Linguist. 2015;5(6):34 https://doi.org/10.5539/ijel.v5n6p34.
31. Almalki M, Fitzgerald G, Clark M. Health care system in Saudi Arabia: an overview. East Mediterr Health J. 2011;17(10):784–93.
32. Ministry of Health (Saudi Arabia). World Health Survey Saudi Arabia (KSAWHS) 2019. Riyadh: Ministry of Health; 2025. Available from: https://www.moh.gov.sa/en/Ministry/Statistics/Population-Health-Indicators/Documents/World-Health-Survey-Saudi-Arabia.pdf
33. Suleiman AK, Ming LC. Transforming healthcare: Saudi Arabia's Vision 2030 healthcare model. J Pharm Policy Pract. 2025;18(1):2449051. https://doi.org/10.1080/20523211.2024.2449051.

Equity and Social Determinants of Health in Saudi Communities

3

Learning Objectives

By the end of this chapter, students will be able to:

1. Define and explain the concepts of health equity, health equality, and social determinants of health (SDH), and differentiate between avoidable and unavoidable health disparities in relation to social justice principles.
2. Analyze the theoretical and conceptual frameworks that underpin health equity.
3. Examine the social, economic, environmental, and cultural factors—such as education, employment, income, gender, housing, food security, and geography—that shape population health outcomes in Saudi Arabia.
4. Evaluate the impact of socioeconomic status, education, and health literacy on the prevalence and management of noncommunicable diseases (NCDs) and other health outcomes within Saudi communities.
5. Discuss how Vision 2030 and the Health Transformation Program address health equity by reforming healthcare delivery, promoting preventative care, and ensuring equitable access to high-quality services across regions and populations.
6. Compare and contrast health equity and equality in the Saudi context, demonstrating how equitable interventions require the adaptation of resources to meet the diverse needs of different population groups.
7. Assess the influence of gender roles, cultural traditions, and regional diversity on health behaviors, access to care, and health-seeking practices.
8. Appraise the role of community health nurses (CHNs) in promoting health equity through advocacy, community assessment, culturally competent care, intersectoral collaboration, and evidence-based policy influence.
9. Integrate global perspectives on SDH to compare how other nations address health disparities, identifying lessons that can inform equitable public health policies and interventions in Saudi Arabia.

R. I. Ashgar, *Community Health Nursing: Principles, Practices, and Perspectives*,
https://doi.org/10.1007/978-3-032-30791-0_3

10. Synthesize knowledge of social determinants, policy frameworks, and nursing practice to design and propose culturally responsive, evidence-based community interventions aimed at reducing health disparities and advancing health equity in Saudi communities.

Health equity, fundamentally, signifies that every individual possesses a just and fair opportunity to achieve their optimal health status, irrespective of their social or economic standing [1]. This concept extends beyond mere access to healthcare services, encompassing the broader societal conditions that influence health outcomes. These conditions, recognized as social determinants of health, are the circumstances in which people are born, grow, live, work, and age [2]. The intricate interplay of these factors necessitates a comprehensive approach, particularly in diverse and rapidly developing nations such as Saudi Arabia, where traditional values and modern advancements converge to shape community well-being. Understanding these determinants is crucial for developing targeted interventions and policies aimed at reducing health disparities and promoting overall population health.

In Saudi Arabia, the epidemiological landscape has shifted from a predominance of communicable diseases to a rise in noncommunicable diseases, underscoring the increasing relevance of socioeconomic determinants and their impact on health equity [3]. The high prevalence of noncommunicable diseases in Saudi Arabia, which accounts for 70% of all deaths, further emphasizes the urgent need to address these underlying socioeconomic factors [3]. This shift necessitates a critical examination of upstream, midstream, and downstream policy measures to improve public health and justice, ensuring that health policy development is informed by a robust assessment of their impact on health equity. This chapter will delve into the multifaceted aspects of health equity and social determinants of health within Saudi communities, exploring the unique cultural and social conditions that influence their advancement.

Conceptualizing Health Equity

A deep understanding of health equity requires an examination of underlying theoretical frameworks that distinguish between avoidable and unavoidable health differences, framing equity as a comparative principle intrinsically linked to social justice and fairness. This perspective posits that disparities arising from systematic, avoidable, and unjust social and economic arrangements are inherently inequitable and demand policy intervention [4, 5]. The World Health Organization defines social determinants of health as the conditions influencing where individuals are born, mature, reside, work, and age, highlighting their pervasive impact on health outcomes [6]. These determinants extend beyond individual choices, encompassing a broad range of environmental and societal factors that profoundly shape health trajectories across the lifespan. For instance, factors such as income, education, occupation, housing, food security, and access to healthcare services directly influence an individual's exposure to health risks and their ability to mitigate them [3]. Furthermore, the upstream/downstream framework illuminates how broader socioeconomic, cultural, and political contexts, alongside public policy, fundamentally influence an individual's socioeconomic position and experiences, thereby impacting health and well-being [7].

In Saudi Arabia, factors such as educational attainment have been shown to significantly influence the prevalence of noncommunicable diseases, with lower education levels correlating with higher disease burdens, particularly among women [3]. This underscores the critical need for a nuanced approach to health equity, distinguishing it from social justice; while health equity focuses on more proximal disparities, social justice addresses the structural issues contributing to disadvantage. Achieving health equity means that every individual should ideally be able to reach their full health potential, free from disadvantage due to social standing or other socially determined circumstances. Thus, health equity is not merely about providing equal access but about providing resources tailored to individual needs, aiming for equitable health outcomes across diverse populations.

Defining Health Equity in a Saudi Context

The Kingdom's Vision 2030, with its emphasis on improving the quality of life and health for all citizens, provides a strategic imperative for addressing health equity through targeted policy and programmatic interventions. This national framework prioritizes the reduction of health disparities by acknowledging the profound impact of social determinants on population health outcomes. It recognizes that systemic changes are essential for ensuring universal access to quality healthcare and addressing avoidable and unfair differences in health outcomes across population groups. Achieving sustainable health equity, therefore, necessitates a holistic approach that simultaneously tackles social inequality and environmental challenges, as these are intrinsically linked in generating health disparities both nationally and globally [8]. This comprehensive strategy aligns with global efforts, such as the Sustainable Development Goals, particularly SDG 3, which advocates for healthy lives and well-being for all, recognizing the interdependence of health with other socioeconomic factors [9]. Saudi Arabia's ongoing health system reforms and investments in healthcare infrastructure, digital health advancements, and public health initiatives demonstrate a commitment to leveraging opportunities while addressing challenges such as the growing prevalence of lifestyle-related diseases. Despite these advancements, ensuring equitable and unbiased access to healthcare services, addressing disparities in health outcomes, and enhancing the overall quality of care across diverse communities still present significant challenges [10].

Distinguishing Health Equity from Health Equality

While often used interchangeably, health equity and health equality are distinct concepts crucial for effective public health interventions. Health equality denotes providing everyone with the same resources and opportunities, whereas health equity focuses on tailoring resources to meet differing needs to achieve comparable health outcomes

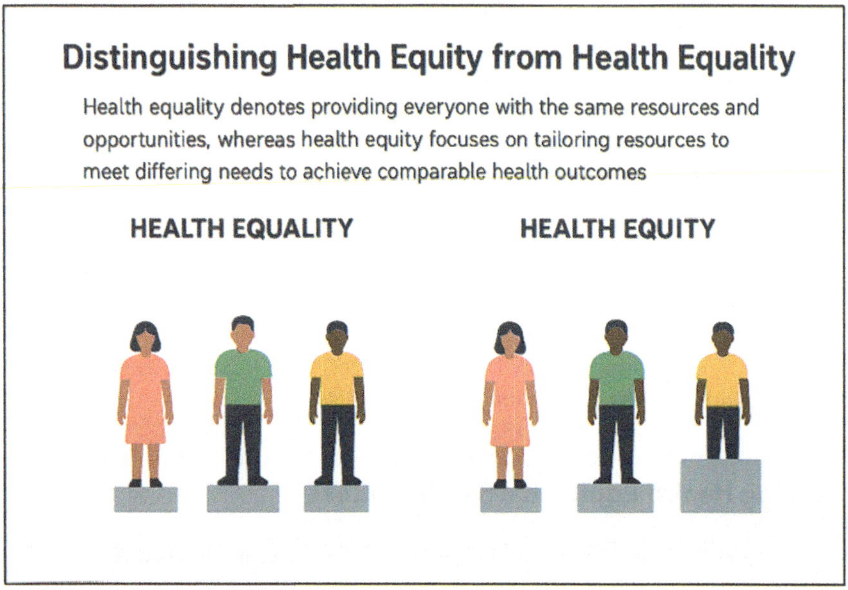

Fig. 3.1 Health equity versus health equality

[11] (see Fig. 3.1). This distinction is particularly salient in the Saudi context, where diverse demographic profiles and varying levels of access to resources necessitate an approach that moves beyond mere equality to achieve genuine equity in health outcomes [10]. For instance, addressing disparities in chronic disease prevalence requires not just equal access to clinics but also targeted programs that account for socioeconomic, educational, and cultural variations influencing health-seeking behaviors and preventative practices. This nuanced approach to health equity acknowledges that equal treatment does not always result in equitable outcomes, especially when existing societal structures disadvantage certain groups. Thus, a critical examination of socioeconomic determinants and their differential impact on various population segments is paramount for developing effective, context-specific interventions that advance health equity. This requires a comprehensive understanding of the intricate interplay between various social, economic, and environmental factors and their collective influence on health outcomes, emphasizing the need for targeted policies and programs that address root causes of disparities. Consequently, the Vision 2030 framework directly addresses these disparities through comprehensive healthcare reforms, including the integration of digital health and telemedicine, to ensure equitable access and quality across all regions [12].

Social Determinants of Health (SDH)

The concept of social determinants of health encompasses the complex, interconnected social and economic factors that profoundly influence individual and community health outcomes, extending beyond direct medical care. These determinants, including factors such as socioeconomic status, education, neighborhood and physical environment, employment, social support networks, and access to healthcare, shape an individual's opportunities and resources for health. In Saudi Arabia, these determinants are particularly critical given the rapid societal transformations and diverse geographical and cultural landscapes, influencing everything from chronic disease prevalence to mental health outcomes [9]. For instance, noncommunicable diseases are significantly influenced by socioeconomic factors, with disparities in prevalence observed across different segments of the population. A higher prevalence of noncommunicable diseases has been noted among women, the elderly (aged 60 and above), and individuals with lower educational attainment, highlighting the pervasive impact of socioeconomic status on health outcomes [3]. These disparities underscore the necessity of developing targeted health interventions and policies that account for the nuanced interplay of socioeconomic factors, cultural practices, and access to resources within the Saudi Arabian context.

Global Perspectives on SDH

Globally, health inequities are deeply rooted in socioeconomic, environmental, and technological factors, further exacerbated by historical influences and contemporary challenges such aspandemics and climate change [13]. The global discourse emphasizes that addressing these complex challenges requires comprehensive strategies focusing on the equitable distribution of resources and opportunities [6]. This international perspective highlights the imperative for nations such as Saudi Arabia to adopt comprehensive, multisectoral approaches that transcend traditional healthcare interventions, integrating social policy with public health initiatives to foster environments conducive to well-being for all citizens.

The WHO Framework for SDH

The World Health Organization framework on the social determinants of health provides a comprehensive model for understanding how various societal factors influence health outcomes, advocating for policies and interventions that address these underlying causes rather than just their manifestations [6]. This framework emphasizes that an individual's social position, which is shaped by the distribution of money, power, and resources at global, national, and local levels, acts as a primary determinant of health inequalities [12]. In the Saudi Arabian context, applying this framework necessitates examining how the rapid economic development, urbanization, and cultural dynamics impact the distribution of health-determining resources and opportunities across different communities and demographic groups.

Key Social Determinants of Health in Saudi Arabia

In Saudi Arabia, several prominent social determinants profoundly influence population health, encompassing socioeconomic status, financial stability, educational attainment, housing and environmental quality, food security, accessibility of healthcare services, gender, and geographical location. These factors, alongside cultural norms and social support networks, significantly shape health behaviors and access to preventative care across diverse Saudi communities.

Socioeconomic Status and Health Outcomes

Socioeconomic status, encompassing income, occupation, and wealth, profoundly dictates an individual's exposure to health risks and access to protective resources [14]. In Saudi Arabia, disparities in socioeconomic status are often reflected in varying health outcomes, with lower-income populations experiencing higher rates of chronic diseases and reduced access to quality healthcare [2]. This pattern is consistent with global observations that link lower socioeconomic status to increased disease burden and mortality rates. Consequently, targeted public health interventions are necessary to address these foundational inequalities. Such interventions and policy adjustments are, therefore, essential to mitigate the health consequences of economic inequality and foster a more equitable distribution of health resources across all segments of society.

Education and Health Literacy

Educational attainment and health literacy are pivotal in shaping individual and community health, directly influencing lifestyle choices, engagement with preventive care, and the effective management of health conditions. Higher educational levels generally correlate with improved health literacy, enabling individuals to better understand health information, navigate healthcare systems, and adopt healthier behaviors [15]. In Saudi Arabia, efforts to enhance health literacy through educational initiatives are crucial for empowering communities to make informed decisions regarding their well-being and to proactively engage in health promotion and disease prevention. These initiatives are vital for addressing the increasing prevalence of chronic diseases and related risk factors, such as insufficient physical activity and unhealthy dietary patterns, observed across the Saudi population.

Employment, Occupation, and Working Conditions

Employment, occupation, and working conditions exert a significant influence on health outcomes by shaping financial stability, exposure to occupational hazards, and opportunities for social engagement. In Saudi Arabia, the rapid economic diversification and expansion of various industries necessitate a critical examination of how different employment sectors contribute to health disparities, particularly concerning workplace safety, job security, and access to health benefits. Furthermore, the nature of employment, ranging from highly skilled professional roles to manual labor, can significantly impact an individual's stress levels, physical activity, and exposure to environmental pollutants, all of which are critical determinants of long-term health [3]. Consequently, addressing these occupational determinants through robust regulatory frameworks and proactive employer-led initiatives is crucial for fostering a healthier workforce and reducing health inequalities. These efforts must also consider the unique demographic and cultural characteristics of the Saudi workforce, including the increasing participation of women and expatriate workers, to ensure equitable and effective health interventions.

Housing, Environment, and Infrastructure

The quality and location of housing, along with access to robust infrastructure and a clean environment, are fundamental determinants of health, directly impacting physical safety, mental well-being, and exposure to environmental risks [16]. In Saudi Arabia, rapid urbanization and development necessitate a critical examination of how varied housing standards and environmental exposures contribute to health disparities across different regions and communities. For instance, inadequate housing can lead to issues such as poor ventilation, overcrowding, and exposure to infectious diseases, while limited access to green spaces can negatively impact mental health and opportunities for physical activity. Furthermore, the spatial distribution of healthcare facilities, transportation networks, and access to nutritious food outlets within different neighborhoods critically shapes health equity by influencing the ease with which individuals can access essential services and resources [17]. The consideration of these factors, including the provision of adequate infrastructure and environmental protections, is vital for mitigating health inequalities and promoting holistic well-being among all residents.

Food Security and Nutrition

Food security and nutrition are paramount to public health, directly influencing growth, development, and resilience against disease. In Saudi Arabia, the prevalence of lifestyle-related diseases, such as noncommunicable diseases, underscores the critical importance of addressing nutritional imbalances and ensuring equitable access to healthy food options. This involves considering the availability, affordability, and cultural appropriateness of nutritious food, as well as the knowledge required to make informed dietary choices. Consequently, robust public health initiatives are essential to counteract the rising incidence of diet-related illnesses by promoting balanced nutritional intake and ensuring widespread access to healthy food options.

Access to Healthcare Services and Quality of Care

Equitable access to comprehensive healthcare services—encompassing preventative, curative, and rehabilitative care—is a fundamental pillar of health equity, and yet, it remains a significant public health challenge in 2024 [18]. This challenge is exacerbated by disparities in chronic disease prevalence, mental health resources, and access to essential medicines, which disproportionately affect vulnerable populations [18]. Therefore, effective public health interventions demand a unified global vision that prioritizes targeted strategies and collaborative efforts to mitigate these deep-seated disparities and foster health security for all populations. Overcoming these multifaceted challenges requires a strategic focus on strengthening primary healthcare infrastructure, improving the distribution of specialized medical professionals, and implementing digital health solutions to overcome geographical barriers. Equally vital is ensuring the quality of care delivered across all healthcare settings, from primary care clinics to tertiary hospitals, encompassing aspects such as patient safety, evidence-based practices, and patient-centered approaches [19]. Saudi Vision 2030 acknowledges the critical role of a robust and accessible healthcare system in achieving national development goals. It emphasizes the need for transformative reforms to enhance efficiency, quality, and equitable access across the Kingdom, thereby underscoring a commitment to addressing existing healthcare disparities and strengthening the foundational elements for a resilient and inclusive health system, particularly in light of global health challenges.

Culture, Traditions, and Social Cohesion

Cultural norms, traditional practices, and the degree of social cohesion within communities significantly influence health behaviors, access to care, and the overall well-being of individuals in Saudi Arabia. Understanding these intricate social determinants is crucial for developing culturally sensitive health interventions and policies that resonate with the local population and effectively address unique health challenges, such as hereditary conditions or traditional healing practices that may impact health-seeking behaviors. Moreover, the preservation of strong family ties and community networks, characteristic of Saudi society, can act as a powerful protective factor against social isolation and mental health issues, necessitating their integration into community health strategies. This understanding of cultural nuances and traditional frameworks is also essential for guiding the development of culturally competent and responsive healthcare services. These services must acknowledge diverse beliefs about health and illness to facilitate better engagement and ultimately improve health outcomes for all community members [20]. Furthermore, where appropriate and evidence-based, integrating traditional knowledge and practices can significantly enhance the relevance and effectiveness of public health initiatives, thereby fostering greater community acceptance and participation.

Gender and Health Disparities

Gender plays a pivotal role in shaping health experiences in Saudi Arabia, where biological differences intersect with sociocultural roles and expectations to produce distinct health profiles and disparities. These inequalities are reflected in the varying prevalence of certain diseases, unequal access to healthcare services, and differences in health-seeking behaviors—all shaped by societal norms and gender-specific responsibilities. Efforts to address these imbalances have included women's empowerment initiatives, which have contributed to greater participation in the healthcare workforce and expanded access to leadership roles [21].

However, gender-specific barriers to healthcare access and utilization persist, significantly influencing the health behaviors of Saudi women [22, 23]. Cultural factors—such as a preference for female physicians—can delay medical consultations and hinder the timely management of chronic conditions, including cardiovascular disease and diabetes [22, 24, 25].

Geographic Location (Urban vs. Rural)

Geographic location significantly influences the accessibility and quality of healthcare services in Saudi Arabia, with rural and remote areas often facing greater challenges. These disparities manifest as fewer healthcare facilities, limited availability of specialized medical professionals, and longer travel times to access essential services, ultimately impacting health outcomes for residents in these regions [3, 26]. Consequently, residents in such areas may experience delays in diagnosis and treatment, exacerbating chronic conditions and reducing overall life expectancy [22]. Addressing these geographical barriers requires targeted interventions, such as expanding telehealth services and establishing mobile clinics, to ensure equitable access to care across the Kingdom. Saudi Vision 2030 recognizes these challenges and aims to bridge the gap through infrastructure development and digital transformation initiatives.

Impact of SDH on Community Health in Saudi Arabia

The intricate interplay of SDH significantly influences the health status of both Saudi and non-Saudi households, revealing pronounced health disparities across different regions. These disparities often manifest as varied prevalence rates of noncommunicable diseases and other health outcomes, directly linked to SDH across different governorates.

Prevalence of Noncommunicable Diseases (NCDs)

Noncommunicable diseases represent a substantial public health burden in Saudi Arabia, with their prevalence significantly influenced by socioeconomic factors and gender [3]. Disparities in healthcare access, cultural norms, and the uneven distribution of facilities contribute to varying NCD prevalence rates across regions [3]. For instance, Saudi women have historically encountered sociocultural barriers to physical activity, such as limited access to exercise facilities and transportation restrictions. This has contributed to a higher prevalence of obesity among them [24]. This gender disparity is further exacerbated by delays in seeking healthcare, which can lead to undiagnosed or untreated cases of chronic conditions, particularly among Saudi women [22].

Regional variations further compound the issue, with areas such as Al-Baha and Ha'il experiencing higher rates of chronic diseases and related mortality compared to more urbanized governorates such as Makkah and Al-Madinah [3, 27]. Socioeconomic factors, including income and educational attainment, also play a critical role, as lower socioeconomic status is consistently associated with a higher burden of NCDs [3, 28]. This association often stems from limited access to nutritious food, reduced engagement in health-promoting behaviors, and insufficient preventative care among disadvantaged populations [29]. Epidemiological data indeed reveal that NCDs account for more than 70% of all deaths in Saudi Arabia, highlighting the critical need to address these underlying social and economic determinants [3]. The Vision 2030 framework directly addresses these health challenges by prioritizing preventative care and disease management to mitigate the impact of NCDs on the population.

Maternal and Child Health Outcomes

Maternal and child health outcomes in Saudi Arabia are significantly influenced by SDH, including socioeconomic status, education, geographic location, and access to quality healthcare services. Recent evidence indicates that the incidence of preterm birth ranges between 4% and 8% of live births, with higher rates reported in rural and peripheral regions [30]. These disparities are often associated with limited access to prenatal and neonatal care, maternal nutritional deficiencies, and variations in health literacy. Although the infant mortality rate (IMR) has declined markedly over the past three decades—reaching about 5 deaths per 1000 live births in 2023 [31]—inequities persist between urban and rural communities. Women and infants in remote areas remain more vulnerable to adverse outcomes due to reduced availability of specialized obstetric and pediatric services. Addressing these gaps through improved healthcare infrastructure, community-based maternal education, and equitable resource allocation is crucial to achieving the national health goals outlined in Saudi Vision 2030 and to promoting sustainable maternal and child health outcomes across all regions of the Kingdom. The Ministry of Health's initiatives, such as expanding primary healthcare centers and enhancing maternal and child health programs, aim to mitigate these disparities and ensure comprehensive care for all mothers and children [27].

Infectious Diseases and Vulnerable Populations

Infectious diseases continue to pose significant challenges to vulnerable populations in Saudi Arabia, with disproportionate impacts on specific demographic groups and regions. Despite a significant overall decline in communicable diseases since 1990, specific infectious agents continue to disproportionately affect migrant workers, pilgrims, and low-income communities [32]. This vulnerability stems from factors such as crowded living conditions and variable access to preventative health services. These populations often face additional barriers, including language difficulties and a lack of awareness about available health resources, which further exacerbate their susceptibility to infectious diseases [33]. The healthcare system's transformation under Vision 2030 aims to address these challenges by restructuring health services to be more comprehensive and effective, incorporating robust surveillance systems and targeted interventions to mitigate the spread of infectious diseases among these vulnerable groups [34].

Moreover, the Hajj and Umrah pilgrimages present unique public health challenges, necessitating stringent infection control measures and rapid response protocols to prevent the widespread transmission of pathogens among millions of international visitors. To manage such mass gatherings, the Ministry of Health has thus prioritized robust emergency preparedness and response strategies, reflecting a key research priority in health agendas [35]. This focus includes dedicated efforts towards understanding individual and community health risks, evaluating outcomes, and appraising interventions, especially within the context of mass gatherings. Such initiatives are critical for ensuring public health security and preventing outbreaks, particularly given the dynamic nature of global travel and population movements. This comprehensive approach aligns with the Kingdom's broader health sector transformation, as outlined in Vision 2030, which emphasizes sustainable funding, equitable access, and continuous improvement in service quality to address public health challenges effectively.

Addressing Health Equity and SDH in Saudi Arabia

Saudi Arabia has proactively implemented a range of policies and initiatives to address health equity and the social determinants of health, reflecting a commitment to national well-being and development [35]. These strategic efforts are primarily guided by the ambitious Vision 2030 framework, which integrates health equity as a core component of its national development plan.

Vision 2030 and Health Transformation Program

Under Vision 2030, the Health Transformation Program specifically aims to restructure the healthcare system to improve efficiency, accessibility, and quality, ensuring that healthcare services are equitably distributed across all regions and socioeconomic strata [20]. This program focuses on shifting from a reactive, hospital-centric model to a proactive, population health-focused approach, emphasizing preventative care and primary healthcare services. A key aspect of this transformation involves leveraging digital health technologies and expanding community-based health initiatives to reach underserved populations and address health disparities effectively.

Role of Governmental and Nongovernmental Organizations

Both governmental bodies and nongovernmental organizations play crucial roles in implementing these health equity initiatives by fostering collaborations and delivering targeted interventions to vulnerable communities [36]. For example, the Saudi Arabian government has invested in establishing public health colleges to cultivate expertise in this domain and has adopted a "Health-in-All Policies" strategy, aligning with WHO recommendations, to ensure that decisions across various sectors consider health implications and promote health equity [37]. Nongovernmental organizations, often working in partnership with governmental agencies, contribute significantly by providing direct services, advocating for marginalized groups, and implementing grassroots programs that address specific social determinants of health at the community level. These concerted efforts are instrumental in translating national health objectives into tangible improvements in community health outcomes, particularly in addressing complex health challenges through collaborative action [38]. This overarching strategy aligns directly with the ambitious goals of Vision 2030, which seeks to transform the Kingdom into a global pioneer by fostering a vibrant society, a thriving economy, and an ambitious nation.

Community-Based Interventions

Community-based interventions are pivotal in operationalizing national objectives by directly addressing health needs within local contexts. These initiatives often empower individuals and families to actively manage their health, fostering informed decision-making and promoting a preventive approach to wellness rather than relying solely on curative models [37]. Facilitated through public–private partnerships, these programs aim to enhance health literacy, promote healthy lifestyles, and ensure equitable access to essential health services, particularly in remote or underserved areas [39]. This approach necessitates robust stakeholder involvement and the integration of diverse activities to ensure policies are both effective and inclusive, ultimately strengthening participation and broadening the knowledge base. Such initiatives are crucial for building resilient communities capable of addressing health disparities, especially in the face of emerging public health challenges, thereby reinforcing the nation's commitment to improving overall population health outcomes.

The Role of Community Health Nursing in Promoting Health Equity

Community health nurses are uniquely positioned to advance health equity through their direct engagement with diverse populations, enabling them to identify and mitigate the social determinants of health at a grassroots level. Their comprehensive approach to healthcare delivery encompasses not only clinical care but also emphasizes prevention, health promotion, and the management of chronic conditions within community settings [40]. This holistic perspective allows community health nurses to act as pivotal liaisons, bridging the gap between healthcare systems and the communities they serve by addressing inequities in access and health outcomes.

Advocacy and Policy Influence

Community health nurses are instrumental in advocating for policy changes that address systemic barriers to health equity, utilizing their direct experiences with vulnerable populations to inform and influence health legislation and resource allocation. They play a crucial role in empowering communities to participate in health policy development, ensuring that interventions are culturally sensitive and responsive to local needs. Their involvement extends to leveraging evidence-based practice and community health data to highlight health disparities, thereby advocating for targeted interventions and resource allocation to underserved communities.

Community Assessment and Needs Identification

Through systematic community health needs assessments, community health nurses meticulously gather data on population health status, social determinants of health, and existing healthcare resources to identify priority areas for intervention. This process involves engaging with community members to understand their perspectives and priorities, ensuring that interventions are tailored to specific local contexts and are culturally appropriate. This deep understanding of community dynamics allows nurses to collaboratively develop interventions that are both effective and sustainable in addressing health inequities.

Health Education and Empowerment

Community health nurses actively engage in designing and delivering tailored health education programs that empower individuals and communities with the knowledge and skills necessary to make informed health decisions and adopt healthy lifestyles. These educational initiatives are crucial for improving health literacy, enabling communities to navigate complex health systems, and fostering self-efficacy in managing personal and communal health challenges.

Intersectoral Collaboration and Partnerships

Community health nurses routinely forge robust partnerships with diverse stakeholders, including governmental bodies, nongovernmental organizations, and community leaders, to develop comprehensive, multipronged strategies aimed at improving health outcomes and fostering sustainable community well-being. This intersectoral collaboration is vital for addressing complex health determinants that extend beyond the healthcare sector, promoting a holistic approach to public health.

Culturally Competent Care Delivery

Community health nurses provide care that is respectful of and responsive to the health beliefs, practices, and cultural and linguistic needs of diverse populations, thereby improving health outcomes and fostering trust within the communities they serve. This culturally competent approach is foundational to achieving health equity, as it ensures that healthcare services are accessible, acceptable, and effective for all individuals, regardless of their background.

References

1. Fairweather J, Jawad A. Overcoming socioeconomic obstacles is important in achieving equity in health care. Saudi Med J. 2024;45(7):749. https://doi.org/10.15537/smj.2024.45.7.20230464.
2. Almujadidi B, Adams AM, AlQuaiz AM, van der Gurp G, Schuster T, Andermann A. Exploring social determinants of health in a Saudi Arabian primary health care setting: the need for a multidisciplinary approach. Int J Equity Health. 2022;21(1):162. https://doi.org/10.1186/s12939-022-01627-2.
3. Al-Hanawi MK. Socioeconomic determinants and inequalities in the prevalence of non-communicable diseases in Saudi Arabia. Int J Equity Health. 2021;20(1):225. https://doi.org/10.1186/s12939-021-01510-6.
4. van den Berg M, Flavel J, Schram A, Friel S, Gesesew HA, Baum F. Social, cultural and political conditions for advancing health equity: examples from eight country case studies (2011–2021). BMJ Glob Health. 2024;9:e015694. https://doi.org/10.1136/bmjgh-2024-015694.
5. Chang WC. A grand plan for health equity. Int J Equity Health. 2025;24(1):36. https://doi.org/10.1186/s12939-025-02536-w.
6. Chelak K, Chakole S. The role of social determinants of health in promoting health equality: a narrative review. Cureus. 2023;15:e33425. https://doi.org/10.7759/cureus.33425.
7. Ray R, Lantz PM, Williams DR. Upstream policy changes to improve population health and health equity: a priority agenda. Milbank Q. 2023;101:20–32. https://doi.org/10.1111/1468-0009.12640.
8. Castro A, Marmot M, Garay J, Negri A, Buss PM. Achieving sustainable health equity. Bull World Health Organ. 2022;100(1):81–9. https://doi.org/10.2471/BLT.21.286523.
9. Alarifi A, Alshahrani N, Jokhdar H, Asiri A. Advancing health through Sustainable Development Goals—Saudi Arabia's mid-journey progress and insights. J Epidemiol Glob Health. 2025;15:48–58. https://doi.org/10.1007/s44197-025-00385-y.
10. Suleiman AK, Ming LC. Transforming healthcare: Saudi Arabia's Vision 2030 healthcare model. J Pharm Policy Pract. 2025;18(1):2449051. https://doi.org/10.1080/20523211.2024.2449051.
11. Stevens A, Neilson M, Rasanathan K, Syed SB, Koller TS. Quality and equity: a shared agenda for universal health coverage. BMJ Glob Health. 2023;8(7):e012561. https://doi.org/10.1136/bmjgh-2023-012561.
12. Marín-Gutiérrez M, Caqueo-Urízar A. The influence of social determinants and 5Cs of positive youthdevelopment on the mental health of Chilean adolescents. BMC Psychol. 2025;13:333. https://doi.org/10.1186/s40359-025-02629-9

13. Rad J. Health inequities: a persistent global challenge from past to future. Int J Equity Health. 2025;24:148. https://doi.org/10.1186/s12939-025-02526-y.
14. González-Rodríguez R, Gandoy-Crego M, Vilaça T. Editorial: social determinants and psychosocial factors that impact on health status. Front Psychol. 2024;15:1405206. https://doi.org/10.3389/fpsyg.2024.1405206.
15. Alshammari M, Duff J, Guilhermino M. Barriers to nurse–patient communication in Saudi Arabia: an integrative review. BMC Nurs. 2019;18:61. https://doi.org/10.1186/s12912-019-0385-4.
16. Buse K, Bestman A, Srivastava S, Marten R, Yangchen S, Nambiar D. What are healthy societies? A thematic analysis of relevant conceptual frameworks. Int J Health Policy Manag. 2023;12:7450. https://doi.org/10.34172/ijhpm.2023.7450.
17. Wick JY. Social determinants of health: how environmental factors affect health. Sr Care Pharm. 2020;35(2):56–61. https://doi.org/10.4140/tcp.n.2020.56.
18. Lucero-Prisno DE, Shomuyiwa DO, Kouwenhoven MBN, Dorji T, Adebisi YA, Odey GO, et al. Top 10 public health challenges for 2024: charting a new direction for global health security. Public Health Chall. 2024;4(1):e70022. https://doi.org/10.1002/puh2.70022.
19. Asmri MA, Almalki M, FitzGerald G, Clark M. The public health care system and primary care services in Saudi Arabia: a system in transition. East Mediterr Health J. 2019;26(4):468–76. https://doi.org/10.26719/emhj.19.049.
20. Al-Anezi. Challenges of healthcare systems in Saudi Arabia to delivering Vision 2030: an empirical study from healthcare workers' perspectives. J Healthc Leadersh. 2025;17:173–87. https://doi.org/10.2147/JHL.S516159.
21. Alzaaqi SM, Sheerah HA, Arafa MA, Alqahtani DM, Al-Qadi SA, Alsalamah HA, et al. Empowering women in the Saudi health sector: challenges, opportunities, and policy interventions. J Epidemiol Glob Health. 2025;15(1):1–12. https://doi.org/10.1007/s44197-025-00361-6.
22. Alissa NA. A cross-sectional study on healthcare-seeking behavior among Saudi women in Riyadh. Sci Rep. 2025;15:93392. https://doi.org/10.1038/s41598-025-93392-9.
23. Habib S, Khan MA, Hamadneh NN. Gender sensitivity in accessing healthcare services: evidence from Saudi Arabia. Sustainability. 2022;14(22):14690. https://doi.org/10.3390/su142214690.
24. AlHabib KF, Batais MA, Almigbal TH, Alshamiri MQ, Altaradi H, Rangarajan S, Yusuf S. Demographic, behavioral, and cardiovascular disease risk factors in the Saudi population: results from the PURE-Saudi study. BMC Public Health. 2020;20(1):1496. https://doi.org/10.1186/s12889-020-09298-w.
25. Alhomayani KM, Bukhary HA, Aljuaid FI, Alotaibi TA, Alqurashi F, Althobaiti K, et al. Gender preferences in healthcare: a study of Saudi patients' physician preferences. Patient Prefer Adherence. 2025;19:295–306. https://doi.org/10.2147/PPA.S494766.
26. Alnahdi S. Households' health status in Saudi Arabia: spatial distribution and association with socioeconomic factors. Res World Econ. 2020;11(3):284–92. https://doi.org/10.5430/rwe.v11n3p284.
27. Alzahrani MS, Alharthi YS, Aljamal JKS, Alarfaj AA, Vennu V, Noweir MD. National and regional rates of chronic diseases and all-cause mortality in Saudi Arabia: analysis of the 2018 Household Health Survey data. Int J Environ Res Public Health. 2023;20(7):5254. https://doi.org/10.3390/ijerph20075254.
28. Alsharif A. Georeferencing of current dental service locations to population census data: identification of underserved areas in Al Madina, Saudi Arabia. SAGE Open. 2020;10(4):2158244020982970. https://doi.org/10.1177/2158244020982970.
29. AlOmar RS, Parslow R, Law G. Development of two socioeconomic indices for Saudi Arabia. BMC Public Health. 2018;18(1):572. https://doi.org/10.1186/s12889-018-5723-z.
30. Almaghaslah E, Ibrahim IA, Al-Zahir SS, Saif A. Prevalence of preterm birth in Saudi Arabia: a systematic review and meta-analysis. Cureus. 2024;16:e74562. https://doi.org/10.7759/cureus.74562.

31. World Bank. Mortality rate, infant (per 1,000 live births) – Saudi Arabia [Internet]. Washington (DC): World Bank; 2025. https://data.worldbank.org/indicator/SP.DYN.IMRT.IN?locations=SA. Accessed 12 Feb 2026.
32. Memish ZA, Alqahtani AS, Alazemi N, Alhamayel NA, Saeedi MF, Abuzinada S, et al. A new era of national guideline development in Saudi Arabia. J Epidemiol Glob Health. 2022;12(4):373–81. https://doi.org/10.1007/s44197-022-00076-y.
33. Salam A. Self-health assessments in Saudi Arabia: directions for an integrated primary healthcare. J Fam Med Prim Care. 2022;11(9):4919–26. https://doi.org/10.4103/jfmpc.jfmpc_2242_21.
34. Alessy SA, Alattas M, Mahmoud MA, Alqarni A, Alghnam S. Population health data in KSA: status, challenges, and opportunities. J Taibah Univ Med Sci. 2022;17(6):1060–68. https://doi.org/10.1016/j.jtumed.2022.06.011.
35. Sheerah HA, Almuzaini Y, Khan A. Public health challenges in Saudi Arabia during the COVID-19 pandemic: a literature review. Healthcare (Basel). 2023;11(12):1757. https://doi.org/10.3390/healthcare11121757.
36. Karlsson LE, Ikonen AL, Alqahtani KM, Andersen PT, Thapa S. Health equity lens embedded in the public health policies of Saudi Arabia: a qualitative document analysis. SAGE Open. 2020;10(4):2158244020962776. https://doi.org/10.1177/2158244020962776.
37. Almalki M, Elamin A, Jabour A, Varghese J, Alotaibi AA, Almalki SM, et al. Awareness of and attitudes toward the public health model among health students in response to Saudi healthcare reform: a cross-sectional study. Front Public Health. 2023;11:1264615. https://doi.org/10.3389/fpubh.2023.1264615.
38. Rahman R, Qattan AMN. Vision 2030 and sustainable development: state capacity to revitalize the healthcare system in Saudi Arabia. Inquiry. 2021;58:0046958020984682. https://doi.org/10.1177/0046958020984682.
39. Hassounah M, Raheel H, Alhefzi M. Digital response during the COVID-19 pandemic in Saudi Arabia. J Med Internet Res. 2020;22(9):e19338. https://doi.org/10.2196/19338.
40. Tushe M, Karagjozi D. The role of community health nursing in improving public health: a global andlocal perspective. Clinical Case Reports and Studies, BioRes Scientia Publishers. 2025;9(2):1-3. https://doi.org/10.59657/2993-0863.brs.25.224

Healthcare System in Saudi Arabia

4

Learning Objectives

By the end of this chapter, students will be able to:

1. Describe the historical evolution of the Saudi healthcare system from traditional healing practices to a modern, government-funded model, highlighting key milestones such as the establishment of the Ministry of Health in 1950.
2. Explain the organizational structure and governance of the Saudi healthcare system, identifying the roles and responsibilities of major entities, including the Ministry of Health, other governmental health sectors, and the private healthcare industry.
3. Differentiate between the primary, secondary, and tertiary levels of healthcare service delivery in Saudi Arabia, explaining their functions, referral pathways, and interconnections within the national health system.
4. Analyze the funding mechanisms and financial sustainability challenges of the Saudi healthcare system, including reliance on government expenditure, the introduction of insurance models, and public–private partnership (PPP) initiatives.
5. Evaluate the key systemic challenges facing Saudi Arabia's healthcare sector—such as workforce imbalances, regional disparities, demographic and epidemiological transitions, and fragmentation of care—and their implications for equitable service delivery.
6. Discuss the Health Sector Transformation Program (HSTP) under Vision 2030, outlining its strategic objectives of improving the quality, efficiency, accessibility, and sustainability of healthcare services across the Kingdom.
7. Examine the government's initiatives toward privatization and value-based healthcare (VBHC), explaining how these reforms aim to improve health outcomes, cost-effectiveness, and patient-centered care.

R. I. Ashgar, *Community Health Nursing: Principles, Practices, and Perspectives*,
https://doi.org/10.1007/978-3-032-30791-0_4

8. Assess the role of digital health transformation in Saudi Arabia—including platforms such as Nafis, Seha Virtual Hospital, Mawid, and Wasfaty—and its potential to enhance care coordination, data integration, and access to services in urban and rural areas.
9. Identify and appraise the strategies for health workforce development and Saudization, focusing on education, training, retention, and professionalization efforts to ensure a sustainable national healthcare workforce.
10. Critically evaluate the monitoring, evaluation, and performance accountability mechanisms established under Vision 2030—such as accreditation, benchmarking, and patient satisfaction systems—and discuss their importance in achieving continuous quality improvement and national health objectives.

The Kingdom of Saudi Arabia (KSA) has undergone profound transformations in its healthcare system over the past few decades. As a high-income nation, Saudi Arabia has prioritized the development of a modern and comprehensive healthcare infrastructure [1]. This chapter provides an overview of the Saudi healthcare system, tracing its historical evolution, analyzing its structure and governance, exploring challenges and reforms, and considering future directions in the context of Saudi Arabia's Vision 2030.

Historical Context and Development

The healthcare system in Saudi Arabia has experienced rapid growth since the discovery of oil in the 1930s [2]. Before this period, healthcare services were limited and primarily traditional in nature, relying on local healers and herbal remedies. Modern medical services began to emerge with the establishment of the Ministry of Health (MOH) in 1950, which marked a pivotal point in the institutionalization of public healthcare services [2].

From the 1970s onward, driven by population growth, the government invested heavily in healthcare infrastructure. Large hospitals, primary healthcare centers (PHCs), and specialized medical cities were constructed across the kingdom. During this era, public healthcare became a constitutional right, and services were offered free of charge to all citizens and public sector expatriates [3, 4].

Structure and Governance

The Saudi Arabian government substantially funds the healthcare system through the Ministry of Health (MOH), allocating a significant portion of its annual budget to healthcare services [2, 5]. This commitment to funding ensures that healthcare remains accessible to all Saudi citizens without direct costs at the point of service. The government's investment in healthcare reflects a broader commitment to social welfare and the well-being of its population [6]. As healthcare costs rise, the government has initiated several strategies aimed at enhancing the efficiency and sustainability of healthcare financing, including exploring public–private partnerships, implementing more efficient resource allocation mechanisms, and strengthening health insurance schemes to promote greater financial responsibility and risk sharing [7, 8].

In addition to the MOH, several other governmental entities provide health services:

- Ministry of Defense (MOD): Operates hospitals for military personnel and their families.
- Ministry of Interior (MOI): Manages healthcare for security forces.
- National Guard Health Affairs: Provides healthcare to National Guard members and their dependents.
- King Faisal Specialist Hospital and Research Centre (KFSHRC): A leading institution for tertiary and quaternary care.
- The private sector, though smaller in scale, plays a growing role, particularly in urban centers. It is regulated by the Saudi Health Council and the Saudi Central Board for Accreditation of Healthcare Institutions (CBAHI) (see Fig. 4.1).

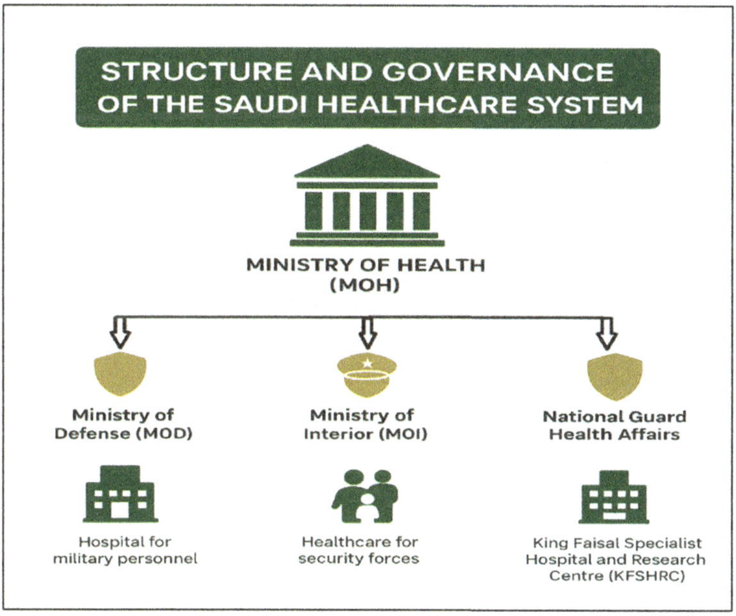

Fig. 4.1 Structure and governance of Saudi healthcare system

Service Delivery

The delivery of healthcare services in Saudi Arabia is structured across a hierarchical system encompassing primary, secondary, and tertiary care levels (see Fig. 4.2), with

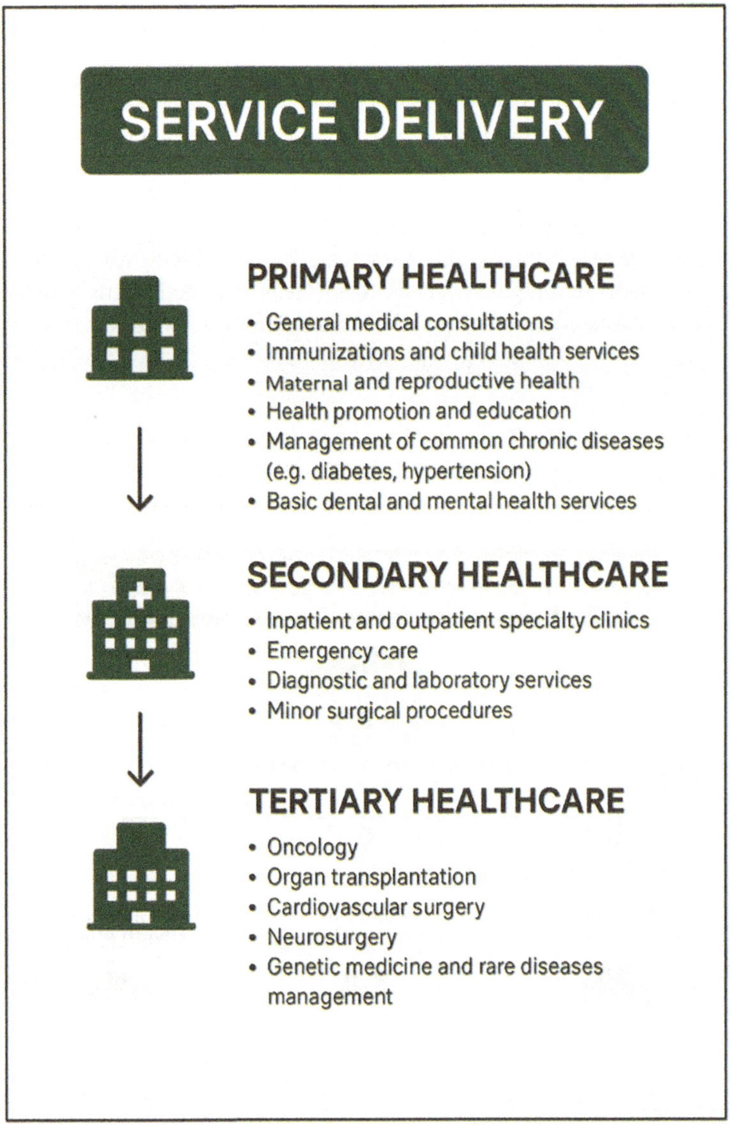

Fig. 4.2 Service delivery in Saudi healthcare system

increasing specialization and complexity at each tier [2, 9]. The Ministry of Health (MOH) is the principal provider, managing the majority of healthcare facilities, while other governmental entities and private providers supplement service delivery, particularly in urban centers.

Primary Healthcare

Primary healthcare centers (PHCs) form the foundation of Saudi Arabia's health service delivery model. The country operates over 2300 PHCs, strategically located to ensure broad geographic coverage, including remote and rural areas [2]. These centers serve as the first point of contact for patients and offer essential services such as:

- General medical consultations
- Immunizations and child health services
- Maternal and reproductive health
- Health promotion and education
- Management of common chronic diseases (e.g., diabetes, hypertension)
- Basic dental and mental health services

The MOH has emphasized the role of PHCs in preventive care, with the goal of reducing the burden on higher levels of the health system. Despite this, PHCs often face challenges related to staffing shortages, inconsistent quality standards, and public perception favoring hospital-based care for even minor conditions [7].

Secondary Healthcare

Secondary care is delivered through general and specialized hospitals distributed across various regions [2]. These facilities provide a broader range of services than PHCs and include:

- Inpatient and outpatient specialty clinics
- Emergency care
- Diagnostic and laboratory services
- Minor surgical procedures

Referrals from PHCs are typically required to access secondary care services, although self-referrals are still common due to the public's preference for hospital-based treatment. A major concern at this level is overcrowding, particularly in urban hospitals, which reflects both high demand and underutilization of PHCs [7].

Tertiary Healthcare

Tertiary care involves highly specialized medical services, often delivered at large referral hospitals or medical cities [2]. Institutions such as King Faisal Specialist Hospital and Research Centre (KFSHRC) and King Abdulaziz Medical Cities provide advanced care including:

- Oncology
- Organ transplantation
- Cardiovascular surgery
- Neurosurgery
- Genetic medicine and rare disease management

Tertiary care, representing the most advanced and experimental treatments, is increasingly becoming available within the Kingdom, reducing the need for patients to travel abroad for care.

Key Challenges

Despite significant progress in expanding and modernizing its healthcare infrastructure, Saudi Arabia's healthcare system faces a range of systemic challenges. These challenges are both structural and emerging, driven by demographic transitions, epidemiological shifts, workforce dynamics, financing and quality pressures, geographic and socioeconomic disparities, fragmentation and coordination of care, and digital transformation and data integration [7, 10, 11]. Addressing these issues is central to achieving the goals set out in Vision 2030 and ensuring the sustainability of the health sector in the long term.

Demographic and Epidemiological Transitions

One of the most pressing challenges is the rapid demographic shift occurring within the Kingdom. The population of Saudi Arabia is not only growing but also aging. The proportion of individuals over the age of 60 is expected to increase substantially over the next two decades, leading to heightened demand for geriatric care, long-term care facilities, and age-related chronic disease management [12].

Coupled with this demographic change is the epidemiological transition from communicable to noncommunicable diseases (NCDs) as the leading causes of morbidity and mortality. Conditions such as diabetes, hypertension, cardiovascular diseases, obesity, and certain types of cancer have become widespread. For instance, the prevalence of diabetes in the adult population exceeds 20%, significantly above the global average [12]. This shift has placed an immense burden on the healthcare system, requiring long-term, resource-intensive management strategies and a shift toward preventive care.

Health Workforce Imbalances

The healthcare workforce in Saudi Arabia is characterized by a high dependence on expatriate professionals, who make up the majority of doctors, nurses, and allied health staff [4, 10, 11]. While expatriates have filled essential gaps in healthcare delivery, their reliance presents vulnerabilities related to continuity of care, cultural and language barriers, and long-term sustainability.

Geographic and Socioeconomic Disparities

Although Saudi Arabia has established an extensive healthcare infrastructure, significant regional disparities remain in both access to and quality of care [4, 7]. While all citizens are entitled to free public healthcare, factors such as health literacy, cultural perceptions of health, geographic isolation, transportation challenges, and inadequate infrastructure hinder equitable utilization of services. Addressing these inequities requires comprehensive policy measures, including workforce redistribution incentives, deployment of mobile healthcare units, and expansion of community-based health outreach programs.

Healthcare Financing and Sustainability

The Saudi healthcare system is heavily reliant on government funding. While this model has supported free access to care for decades, it is increasingly viewed as financially unsustainable in the face of rising healthcare costs, population growth, and economic diversification efforts.

The cost burden of chronic diseases, high-tech interventions, and tertiary care services continues to grow [6]. Moreover, inefficiencies such as unnecessary hospital visits, overutilization of services, and a weak referral system exacerbate financial strain. As a result, the government has initiated reforms aimed at introducing insurance-based financing, public–private partnerships (PPPs), and value-based healthcare models to enhance cost-efficiency and sustainability [13–15].

Fragmentation and Coordination of Care

The healthcare system in Saudi Arabia has historically exhibited a fragmented structure, characterized by the operation of multiple governmental agencies and private sector providers in isolated and uncoordinated frameworks. This has resulted in duplication of services, inefficiencies in resource allocation, and difficulties in achieving continuity of care. Patients often bypass primary care services, directly accessing secondary or tertiary hospitals, which increases costs and reduces the effectiveness of primary-level interventions.

To address this, the government is implementing structural reforms, including the regional health cluster model, which aims to integrate care across levels and institutions [16, 17]. However, establishing seamless referral pathways, data sharing systems, and collaborative clinical governance remains a complex and ongoing task.

Quality and Safety of Healthcare Services

While substantial investments have been made to improve healthcare infrastructure, concerns remain regarding the quality and consistency of service delivery [1]. Variability in clinical practice, gaps in patient safety protocols, limited adoption of evidence-based guidelines, and occasional medical errors have prompted increased regulatory scrutiny.

The Saudi Central Board for Accreditation of Healthcare Institutions (CBAHI) plays a key role in enforcing quality standards, yet adherence can vary significantly, particularly between urban and rural facilities or between public and private providers. Continuous quality improvement, robust monitoring mechanisms, and investment in clinical training are needed to ensure safe and effective care across the system.

Digital Transformation and Data Integration

Although Saudi Arabia has made notable advances in digital health infrastructure, challenges remain in fully integrating these technologies into everyday clinical practice. The lack of interoperability among Electronic Health Records (EHRs), limited digital literacy among healthcare professionals, and uneven access to the internet and IT infrastructure in some regions hinder the full potential of digital health solutions [18, 19]. Initiatives such as Nafis (national health information exchange) and Seha (telemedicine platform) are steps in the right direction.

Recent Reforms and Vision 2030

The healthcare sector in Saudi Arabia is currently undergoing a transformative phase, guided by the strategic framework of Vision 2030, which aims to diversify the national economy and enhance the efficiency and sustainability of public services, including healthcare [15]. Central to this transformation is the Health Sector Transformation Program (HSTP), launched as part of Vision 2030 to ensure the delivery of high-quality, accessible, and financially sustainable healthcare services.

Health Sector Transformation Program (HSTP)

The Health Sector Transformation Program, launched in 2020, represents the primary mechanism through which healthcare reform is being operationalized under Vision 2030. Its main goals include:

- Improving healthcare access and quality
- Enhancing efficiency in health service delivery
- Promoting preventive care and public health
- Achieving financial sustainability
- Empowering patients and enhancing the patient experience

To meet these objectives, the program focuses on institutional restructuring, technology adoption, investment in human capital, and promotion of the private sector's role [15].

Institutional Restructuring and Governance Reform

A key reform involves redefining the role of the Ministry of Health (MOH). Traditionally, the MOH has served as both a provider and regulator of healthcare services. Under the reform agenda, the MOH is transitioning into a regulatory and policymaking body, while service delivery is being decentralized to newly established regional health clusters [2, 8, 16].

These health clusters are semi-autonomous entities tasked with managing all health services within a specific geographic area. The goal is to encourage local decision-making, foster accountability, and create integrated care networks that operate more efficiently and are responsive to community needs.

Privatization and Public–Private Partnerships (PPPs)

In line with Vision 2030's economic diversification strategy, the Saudi government is actively promoting privatization and public–private partnerships within the healthcare sector [14]. The objectives include:

- Reducing the financial burden on the state
- Encouraging innovation and competition
- Increasing the role of the private sector in service provision, hospital operations, and health insurance

Key initiatives include the transfer of public hospitals to private operators, the outsourcing of non-clinical services (e.g., diagnostics, catering), and incentives for private investment in underserved regions. The establishment of the National Center for Privatization (NCP) facilitates these processes by ensuring regulatory clarity and supporting project development.

Implementation of Value-Based Healthcare

A major philosophical and operational shift under Vision 2030 is the move toward value-based healthcare (VBHC). This model emphasizes health outcomes relative to the cost of delivering those outcomes, rather than focusing on service volume.

The implementation of VBHC involves:

- Developing national performance indicators tied to patient outcomes
- Encouraging provider competition based on quality rather than quantity
- Aligning payment models (e.g., bundled payments, pay-for-performance)
- Enhancing transparency through public reporting of healthcare performance

This approach is expected to improve the quality of care, reduce waste, and better align healthcare services with patient needs and expectations [8].

Expansion of Preventive and Public Health Services

Historically, the Saudi healthcare system has been more reactive than preventive, heavily focused on curative and hospital-based services. Vision 2030 emphasizes a proactive public health model, with expanded investment in:

- Community-based health promotion
- Early detection and screening programs for chronic diseases
- National campaigns to reduce risk factors such as obesity, tobacco use, and sedentary lifestyles
- Immunization and communicable disease control

The MOH and related agencies are working to build public health capacity, improve surveillance systems, and integrate preventive care into PHC services [15].

Digital Health Transformation

Digital transformation is a cornerstone of Vision 2030's health reform strategy. Saudi Arabia is investing heavily in eHealth infrastructure, with aims to improve service efficiency, enhance clinical decision-making, and empower patients through better access to health information [19].

Major digital health initiatives include:

- **Nafis:** A national health information exchange platform for seamless sharing of medical records across providers.
- **Seha Virtual Hospital:** A telehealth platform offering remote consultations, e-clinics, and access to specialist care for patients in remote areas.
- **Mawid:** An electronic appointment system for primary healthcare centers.
- **Wasfaty:** A nationwide e-prescription platform connecting doctors, patients, and pharmacies.
- **Tabaud and Tawakkalna Apps:** Developed during the COVID-19 pandemic to support contact tracing, testing, and vaccine registration.

These tools have contributed to improved care coordination, reduced unnecessary visits, and enhanced pandemic response capabilities.

Workforce Development and Saudization

Human resource development is essential to the success of healthcare reforms. Vision 2030 emphasizes increasing the proportion of Saudi nationals in the health workforce, particularly in roles currently dominated by expatriates [10, 11].

Strategies to support this goal include:

- Expanding medical and nursing education programs
- Establishing partnerships with international institutions for training and accreditation
- Enhancing professional development opportunities
- Improving working conditions and career incentives for healthcare workers

Monitoring, Evaluation, and Performance Accountability

To ensure reform implementation is effective and transparent, the government has introduced mechanisms for monitoring and evaluation, including:

- National performance metrics and benchmarking
- Accreditation and quality assurance through the Saudi Central Board for Accreditation of Healthcare Institutions (CBAHI)
- Patient satisfaction surveys and feedback systems
- Audits and financial oversight of privatized services

These mechanisms are designed to foster a culture of continuous improvement and align healthcare delivery with strategic national objectives [9, 15].

References

1. Mani Z, Goniewicz K. Transforming healthcare in Saudi Arabia: a comprehensive evaluation of Vision 2030's impact. Sustainability. 2024;16(8):3277. https://doi.org/10.3390/su16083277.
2. Ministry of Health (Saudi Arabia). Ministry structure [Internet]. Riyadh: Ministry of Health; 2024 [cited 2026 Feb 13]. Available from: https://www.moh.gov.sa/en/Ministry/Structure/Pages/default.aspx
3. Mufti M. Healthcare development strategies in the Kingdom of Saudi Arabia. New York (NY): Springer; 2000.
4. Yousef L, AlAngari D, AlShehri R, AlSharif B, Bayameen O, Alnemer Z. Healthcare transformation journey in the Eastern Region of Saudi Arabia: an overview, challenges and lessons learned. J Med Life. 2023;16(4):583–92. https://doi.org/10.25122/jml-2023-0010.
5. Ministry of Health (Saudi Arabia). Strategies, policies and SLA [Internet]. Riyadh: Ministry of Health; 2025 [cited 2026 Feb 13]. Available from: https://www.moh.gov.sa/en/Ministry/About/Strategy_Policies_SLA/Pages/default.aspx
6. World Bank. Current health expenditure (% of GDP) – Saudi Arabia [Internet]. Washington (DC): World Bank; 2025 [cited 2026 Feb 13]. Available from: https://data.worldbank.org/indicator/SH.XPD.CHEX.GD.ZS?locations=SA
7. Al-Anezi FM. Challenges of healthcare systems in Saudi Arabia to delivering Vision 2030: an empirical study from healthcare workers' perspectives. J Healthc Leadersh. 2025;17:173–87. https://doi.org/10.2147/JHL.S516159.
8. Alasiri AA, Mohammed V. Healthcare transformation in Saudi Arabia: an overview since the launch of Vision 2030. Health Serv Insights. 2022;15:11786329221121214. https://doi.org/10.1177/11786329221121214.
9. Suleiman AK, Ming LC. Transforming healthcare: Saudi Arabia's Vision 2030 healthcare model. J Pharm Policy Pract. 2025;18(1):2449051. https://doi.org/10.1080/20523211.2024.2449051.
10. Albejaidi F, Nair KS. Building the health workforce: Saudi Arabia's challenges in achieving Vision 2030. Int J Health Plann Manag. 2019;34(4):e1405–16. https://doi.org/10.1002/hpm.2861.
11. Elsheikh AS, Alqurashi AM, Wahba MA, Hodhod TE. Healthcare workforce in Saudi Arabia under Saudi Vision 2030. J Health Inform Dev Ctries. 2018;12(1). Available from: https://www.jhidc.org/index.php/jhidc
12. World Health Organization. World Health Survey Saudi Arabia 2019 [Internet]. Geneva: WHO; 2019 [cited 2026 Feb 13]. Available from: https://www.moh.gov.sa/en/Ministry/Statistics/Population-Health-Indicators/Documents/World-Health-Survey-Saudi-Arabia.pdf
13. Almalki A, Al-Hanawi M. Public–private partnerships and collaboration in the health sector in the Kingdom of Saudi Arabia: a qualitative study. Glob J Health Sci. 2018;10(6):10–8. https://doi.org/10.5539/gjhs.v10n6p10.
14. Khan C, Nasrulddin V. Privatization, corporatization, and public–private partnership in the Kingdom of Saudi Arabia. Health Serv Insights. 2022;15:11786329221104240. https://doi.org/10.1177/11786329221104240.
15. Vision 2030 (Saudi Arabia). Health Sector Transformation Program [Internet]. Riyadh: Vision 2030; 2025 [cited 2026 Feb 13]. Available from: https://www.vision2030.gov.sa/en/explore/programs/health-sector-transformation-program
16. Health Holding Company (Saudi Arabia). Health clusters [Internet]. Riyadh: Health Holding Company; 2025 [cited 2026 Feb 13]. Available from: https://www.health.sa/en/clusters
17. Ministry of Health (Saudi Arabia). Corporatization of healthcare facilities [Internet]. Riyadh: Ministry of Health; 2024 [cited 2026 Feb 13]. Available from: https://www.moh.gov.sa/en/Ministry/vro/Corporatization/Pages/default.aspx
18. Alomari A, Soh B. Influences and barriers in the Kingdom of Saudi Arabia affecting technology adoption in healthcare: a review. Int J Comput Sci Netw Secur. 2023;23(6):59–67. https://doi.org/10.22937/IJCSNS.2023.23.6.8.
19. Masmali F, Miah S. Internet of Things adoption for Saudi healthcare services. Pac Asia J Assoc Inf Syst. 2021;13:113–130. https://doi.org/10.17705/1pais.13306.

5 Innovations and Technology in Community Health Nursing

Learning Objectives

By the end of this chapter, students will be able to:

1. Describe the major technological innovations transforming community health nursing, including telehealth, electronic health records (EHRs), mobile health (mHealth), and data analytics, and their relevance to modern healthcare delivery.
2. Explain the principles, applications, and benefits of telehealth technologies in enhancing healthcare accessibility, continuity of care, and patient engagement within the community and underserved populations.
3. Analyze the role of electronic health records (EHRs) in improving care coordination, documentation accuracy, public health surveillance, and patient participation in community health settings.
4. Evaluate the potential of mobile health (mHealth) technologies to promote preventive health behaviors, chronic disease management, and health education across diverse community populations.
5. Discuss the application of data analytics in community health nursing for identifying population health trends, predicting disease outbreaks, evaluating interventions, and supporting evidence-based decision-making.
6. Assess the challenges associated with the adoption of digital health technologies—including privacy, security, interoperability, and the digital divide—and propose strategies to mitigate these barriers.
7. Demonstrate understanding of how current and emerging trends, such as artificial intelligence, interprofessional collaboration, and sustainability initiatives, are shaping the future of community health nursing practice.

R. I. Ashgar, *Community Health Nursing: Principles, Practices, and Perspectives*,
https://doi.org/10.1007/978-3-032-30791-0_5

8. Integrate concepts of technological innovation with the ethical, legal, and professional responsibilities of community health nurses in delivering safe, equitable, and patient-centered care.
9. Critically appraise the impact of Vision 2030 and global health policies on advancing digital transformation and innovation in community health nursing practice.
10. Design evidence-informed strategies for incorporating technological tools into community-based health programs to improve health outcomes and promote health equity.

Telehealth Applications

Telehealth applications have emerged as a transformative force in community health nursing, offering innovative solutions to enhance healthcare delivery and accessibility [1, 2]. The integration of telehealth technologies enables healthcare professionals to extend their reach beyond traditional clinical settings, thus bridging the gap between providers and patients, especially in underserved areas [3]. This expansion of healthcare services is particularly crucial in community health nursing, where the focus is on promoting health and preventing disease within populations.

Telehealth encompasses a wide range of applications, including telemedicine, remote patient monitoring, and mobile health, each contributing uniquely to community health. Telemedicine, a core component of telehealth, facilitates real-time interactions between healthcare providers and patients through video conferencing and other digital communication tools. This capability not only provides immediate access to medical consultations but also supports continuity of care for patients with chronic conditions who require regular monitoring [4, 5]. Remote patient monitoring (RPM) is another critical telehealth application that empowers patients to manage their health conditions more effectively. By utilizing various digital devices, patients can track vital signs and other health metrics, which are then transmitted to healthcare providers for analysis. This continuous flow of health data allows for timely interventions and personalized care plans, significantly improving patient outcomes. RPM is especially beneficial for managing chronic diseases such as diabetes, hypertension, and heart failure, where ongoing monitoring is essential for effective management [6]. Mobile health, or mHealth, further expands the scope of telehealth by leveraging the widespread use of smartphones and mobile devices to deliver health services and information. mHealth applications provide a convenient platform for health education, appointment scheduling, medication reminders, and lifestyle tracking. These tools are instrumental in fostering patient engagement and self-management, key components of effective community health nursing [7, 8].

The adoption of telehealth applications in community health nursing is driven by several factors, including advances in technology, increasing healthcare costs, and the need for more efficient healthcare delivery models. Telehealth offers a cost-effective solution to these challenges by reducing the need for physical infrastructure and minimizing travel expenses for both patients and providers [1, 9]. Moreover, telehealth enhances the capacity of community health nurses (CHNs) to deliver care to a larger population, addressing the growing demand for healthcare services.

However, the implementation of telehealth in community health nursing is not without challenges. Issues such as data security, patient privacy, and the digital divide pose significant barriers to widespread adoption [10–13]. Ensuring the confidentiality and integrity of health information is paramount, as breaches could undermine patient trust and the effectiveness of telehealth services. Additionally, disparities in access to technology and internet connectivity can limit the reach of telehealth applications, particularly in rural or low-income communities. Despite these challenges, the potential benefits of telehealth applications in community health nursing are undeniable. By facilitating timely access to healthcare services, improving patient engagement, and supporting proactive health management, telehealth holds the promise of enhancing the quality and efficiency of community health nursing [9, 14]. As technology continues to evolve, it is essential for healthcare systems and policymakers to address the barriers to telehealth adoption, ensuring that its benefits are accessible to all members of the community.

Electronic Health Records

The integration of electronic health records (EHRs) into community health nursing represents a significant advancement in the management and delivery of healthcare services. EHRs are digital versions of patients' paper charts and are real-time, patient-centered records that make information available instantly and securely to authorized users. These records are designed to contain and share information from all providers involved in a patient's care, thus ensuring continuity and coordination. In community health nursing, the implementation of EHRs facilitates the seamless exchange of health information among healthcare providers, patients, and other stakeholders. This exchange is crucial in providing comprehensive care that is both efficient and effective. By having access to a patient's complete medical history, healthcare providers can make more informed decisions, reduce the risk of errors, and improve patient outcomes [15, 16].

One of the primary benefits of EHRs in community health nursing is the enhancement of care coordination. Patients often receive care from multiple providers, and EHRs ensure that all parties have access to the same information. This coordinated approach is especially important in managing chronic conditions, where consistent monitoring and adjustments to treatment plans are necessary [4, 7, 8]. EHRs support this by providing a platform for tracking patient progress, medication management, and scheduling follow-up appointments.

Moreover, EHRs contribute to the improvement of public health outcomes by enabling the collection and analysis of health data on a larger scale [15]. Public health officials can use aggregated data from EHRs to identify trends, track disease outbreaks, and plan interventions. This data-driven approach allows for more targeted and timely public health responses, ultimately enhancing community health.

In addition to improving care coordination and public health outcomes, EHRs also play a role in patient engagement [5, 16]. Patients can access their own health records, which empowers them to take an active role in their healthcare. This transparency helps patients understand their conditions and treatments better, leading to improved adherence to medical advice and treatment regimens.

However, the implementation of EHRs in community health settings is not without challenges. Issues such as data privacy, system interoperability, and the need for adequate training for healthcare providers are significant considerations. Ensuring the security of patient data is paramount, as breaches can undermine trust and compromise patient confidentiality [6, 10]. Therefore, robust security measures and compliance with regulations are essential.

Interoperability, or the ability of different EHR systems to communicate with one another, is another critical challenge. Without interoperability, the full benefits of EHRs cannot be realized, as information cannot be seamlessly shared across different healthcare settings. Efforts are ongoing to standardize EHR systems to overcome these barriers.

Training and support for healthcare providers are crucial for the successful implementation of EHRs [15]. Providers must be proficient in using these systems to maximize their benefits and minimize disruptions to clinical workflows. Continuous education and support are necessary to keep pace with technological advancements and ensure that EHRs enhance rather than hinder healthcare delivery. In conclusion, while challenges remain, the adoption of EHRs in community health nursing holds great promise for improving healthcare quality, efficiency, and outcomes. By facilitating better communication, enhancing data collection, and empowering patients, EHRs are a pivotal component in advancing community health.

Mobile Health Technologies

Mobile health technologies represent a transformative aspect of modern healthcare, particularly in the context of community health nursing. These technologies encompass a broad range of devices and applications designed to support health services and information via mobile platforms. The proliferation of smartphones and wearable devices has catalyzed the adoption of mobile health technologies, offering innovative solutions for health monitoring, disease management, and patient education [2].

One of the primary advantages of mobile health technologies is their ability to enhance access to healthcare services, especially in underserved areas. Mobile devices can bridge the gap between patients and healthcare providers, facilitating remote consultations and telemedicine services. This is particularly beneficial in rural or remote communities where healthcare resources are limited. By leveraging mobile health technologies, healthcare professionals can provide timely advice, monitor patient conditions in real-time, and adjust treatment plans as necessary, thereby improving patient outcomes. Furthermore, mobile health applications are instrumental in chronic disease management. They offer functionalities such as medication reminders, symptom tracking, and personalized health tips, empowering patients to take an active role in managing their health [8]. For individuals with chronic conditions such as diabetes or hypertension, these applications can provide critical insights into their health patterns, enabling them to make informed decisions about their lifestyle and treatment. Additionally, data collected from these applications can be shared with healthcare providers, facilitating more informed clinical decisions and fostering a collaborative approach to healthcare.

In the realm of community health education, mobile health technologies serve as powerful tools for disseminating information. They can deliver tailored health education materials to individuals, promoting awareness and understanding of various health topics. Interactive features such as quizzes, videos, and forums can engage users and reinforce learning, making health education more accessible and engaging. This is particularly important in promoting preventive health behaviors and reducing the incidence of communicable and non-communicable diseases within communities.

Despite their numerous benefits, the implementation of mobile health technologies also presents challenges. Privacy and security concerns are paramount, as sensitive health data is transmitted and stored on mobile platforms. Ensuring the confidentiality and integrity of this data is critical to maintaining patient trust and complying with regulatory standards. Additionally, there is a need for ongoing evaluation and validation of mobile health applications to ensure their effectiveness and reliability. Healthcare providers must be equipped with the necessary skills and knowledge to integrate these technologies into their practice effectively. Moreover, there are disparities in access to mobile health technologies, often influenced by socioeconomic factors [12, 13]. Addressing these disparities is crucial to ensuring equitable access to healthcare services. Initiatives aimed at increasing digital literacy and providing affordable mobile devices can help bridge this digital divide, enabling more individuals to benefit from mobile health innovations.

In conclusion, mobile health technologies hold significant promise for enhancing community health nursing. By improving access to healthcare, supporting chronic disease management, and facilitating health education, these technologies can play a pivotal role in advancing public health outcomes. As the landscape of mobile health continues to evolve, it is essential for healthcare professionals to stay abreast of technological advancements and integrate them into their practice to maximize their potential benefits.

Data Analytics in Health

The integration of data analytics into health systems has transformed the landscape of community health nursing. By leveraging data-driven insights, healthcare professionals can now enhance patient outcomes, optimize resource allocation, and implement more effective public health interventions. Data analytics in health encompasses a wide array of techniques, including statistical analysis, predictive modeling, and machine learning, which collectively empower nurses to make informed decisions based on empirical evidence [2, 3].

In the realm of community health, data analytics plays a pivotal role in identifying health trends and patterns. By analyzing large datasets, CHNs can discern prevalent health issues within specific populations, such as the incidence of chronic diseases, vaccination rates, and environmental health risks. This capability allows for the proactive identification of at-risk groups, enabling targeted interventions that can mitigate the onset of disease and promote overall health. Moreover, data analytics facilitates the evaluation of health programs and policies. By employing sophisticated analytical tools, healthcare professionals can assess the efficacy of interventions, ensuring that resources are utilized efficiently and effectively. For instance, by analyzing patient outcomes and healthcare utilization data, nurses can determine the impact of preventive measures, such as health education campaigns or vaccination drives, thereby refining future strategies to better serve the community.

Predictive analytics, a subset of data analytics, is particularly valuable in forecasting potential health crises and allocating resources accordingly [2]. By analyzing historical and real-time data, predictive models can anticipate outbreaks of infectious diseases or identify potential healthcare shortages. This foresight enables community health systems to prepare adequately, ensuring that necessary measures are in place to address emerging health threats promptly. Furthermore, data analytics enhances patient-centered care by personalizing treatment plans. Through the analysis of individual health data, nurses can tailor interventions to meet the specific needs of patients, thereby improving adherence to treatment regimens and enhancing patient satisfaction. This personalized approach not only fosters better health outcomes but also empowers patients to take an active role in managing their health.

Despite its numerous benefits, the integration of data analytics in health is not without challenges. Issues such as data privacy, security, and the ethical use of health data must be carefully navigated to maintain patient trust and uphold professional standards. As community health nursing continues to evolve, ongoing education and training in data analytics will be essential to equip nurses with the skills necessary to harness the full potential of data-driven healthcare. In conclusion, data analytics represents a transformative force in community health nursing. By enabling the analysis of complex health data, it provides invaluable insights that drive improvements in patient care and public health outcomes. As the healthcare landscape continues to evolve, the integration of data analytics will undoubtedly play an increasingly critical role in shaping the future of community health nursing, ensuring that it remains responsive to the needs of the populations it serves.

Future Trends

The landscape of community health nursing is evolving rapidly, driven by various technological, societal, and policy changes. One significant trend is the integration of advanced technologies into healthcare practices. The rise of telehealth and mobile health applications is transforming how CHNs deliver care, allowing for real-time monitoring and communication with patients. These technologies enable nurses to reach underserved populations, thereby addressing disparities in access to healthcare services. Furthermore, the use of electronic health records (EHRs) is becoming increasingly prevalent, enhancing the ability of nurses to coordinate care and track patient outcomes over time.

Another important trend is the growing emphasis on population health management. This approach focuses on improving the health outcomes of entire communities rather than just individual patients. CHNs play a crucial role in this model by implementing preventive measures, health education, and chronic disease management programs. By analyzing data and identifying at-risk populations, nurses can develop targeted interventions that address specific health needs within the community.

The role of community health nursing is also expanding in response to the increasing prevalence of chronic diseases. As the population ages and lifestyle-related health issues become more common, there is a greater need for nurses to manage chronic conditions such as diabetes, hypertension, and obesity. This shift requires CHNs to develop new skills and knowledge to effectively educate and support patients in managing their health.

Moreover, there is a growing recognition of the social determinants of health and their impact on community well-being. Factors such as socioeconomic status, education, and environment significantly influence health outcomes. CHNs are increasingly involved in addressing these determinants by advocating for policy changes, collaborating with community organizations, and developing programs that promote health equity.

Interprofessional collaboration is another trend shaping the future of community health nursing. Nurses are working alongside other healthcare professionals, social workers, educators, and policymakers to create comprehensive care plans that address the complex needs of communities. This collaborative approach enhances the quality of care and ensures that all aspects of a patient's well-being are considered.

Finally, there is an increased focus on sustainability and environmental health. CHNs are becoming more involved in initiatives aimed at reducing environmental hazards and promoting sustainable practices. By educating communities about the links between the environment and health, nurses can help mitigate the effects of climate change and other environmental issues on public health. In summary, the future of community health nursing is marked by innovation, collaboration, and a holistic approach to health care. By embracing these trends, CHNs can continue to play a vital role in improving the health and well-being of populations worldwide.

References

1. Badil. The role of telehealth in transforming nursing care: opportunities and challenges. NURSEARCHER (J Nurs Midwifery Sci). 2023;3(2):1. https://doi.org/10.54393/nrs.v3i02.59.
2. McBride S, Tietze M. Nursing informatics for the advanced practice nurse: patient safety, quality, outcomes, and interprofessionalism. 3rd ed. Cham: Springer; 2022.
3. McGonigle D, Mastrian K. Nursing informatics and the foundation of knowledge. 5th ed. Burlington (MA): Jones & Bartlett Learning; 2021.

4. Bashshur RL, Shannon GW, Smith BR, Alverson DC, Antoniotti N, Barsan WG, et al. The empirical foundations of telemedicine interventions for chronic disease management. Telemed J E Health. 2014;20(9):769–800. https://doi.org/10.1089/tmj.2014.9981.
5. Ezeamii VC, Okobi OE, Wambai-Sani H, Perera GS, Zaynieva S, Okonkwo CC, et al. Revolutionizing healthcare: how telemedicine is improving patient outcomes and expanding access to care. Cureus. 2024;16(7):e63881 https://doi.org/10.7759/cureus.63881.
6. Feldman SS, Buchalter S, Hayes LW. Health information technology in healthcare quality and patient safety: literature review. JMIR Med Inform. 2018;6(2):e10264 https://doi.org/10.2196/10264.
7. Fan KZY. Mobile health technology: a novel tool in chronic disease management. Intell Med. 2022;2(1). https://doi.org/10.1016/j.imed.2021.06.003.
8. Mamidi S. Mobile health apps for chronic disease management. J Health Stat Rep. 2022;1(1):1–3. https://doi.org/10.47363/JHSR/2022(1)E104.
9. Chang H, Choi JY, Shim J, Kim M, Choi M. Benefits of information technology in healthcare: artificial intelligence, Internet of Things, and personal health records. Healthc Inform Res. 2023;29(4):323–33.
10. Galavi Z, Montazeri M, Ahmadian L. Barriers and challenges of using health information technology in home care: a systematic review. Int J Health Plann Manage. 2022;37(5):2542–68. https://doi.org/10.1002/hpm.3492.
11. Kruse CS, Stein A, Thomas H, Kaur H. The use of electronic health records to support population health: a systematic review of the literature. J Med Syst. 2018;42(11):214. https://doi.org/10.1007/s10916-018-1075-6.
12. Palacholla RS, Fischer N, Coleman A, Agboola S, Kirley K, Felsted J, et al. Provider- and patient-related barriers to and facilitators of digital health technology adoption for hypertension management: scoping review. JMIR Cardio. 2019;3(1):e11951 https://doi.org/10.2196/11951.
13. Sittig DF, Wright A, Coiera E, Magrabi F, Ratwani R, Bates DW, Singh H. Current challenges in health information technology-related patient safety. Health Inform J. 2020;26(1):181–9. https://doi.org/10.1177/1460458218814893.
14. Sockolow PS, Bowles KH, Topaz M, Koru G, Hellesø R, O'Connor M, Bass EJ. The time is now: informatics research opportunities in home health care. Appl Clin Inform. 2021;12(1):100–6. https://doi.org/10.1055/s-0040-172.
15. Darvish A, Bahramnezhad F, Keyhanian S, Navidhamidi M. The role of nursing informatics on promoting quality of health care and the need for appropriate education. Glob J Health Sci. 2014;6(6):11–8. https://doi.org/10.5539/gjhs.v6n6p11.
16. Hess S, Alper C. Nursing informatics: the vital nursing link between technology and patient care. HCA Healthc J Med. 2024;5(5):513–6. https://doi.org/10.36518/2689-0216.2003.

Community Assessment and Practice Settings 6

Learning Objectives

By the end of this chapter, students will be able to:

1. Explain the fundamental concepts of community structure, function, and dynamics, and how these influence population health and community nursing practice.
2. Describe and apply systematic approaches to conducting a comprehensive community health assessment, including data collection, analysis, and interpretation of social, economic, and environmental determinants of health.
3. Develop a community health diagnosis based on assessed needs, available resources, and identified health problems, demonstrating the ability to prioritize issues using evidence-based criteria.
4. Design appropriate planning and implementation strategies that align with community needs, nursing roles, and public health principles to promote, maintain, and restore health.
5. Evaluate community health programs and interventions by applying principles of outcome measurement, effectiveness assessment, and continuous quality improvement.
6. Utilize feedback mechanisms to refine community health plans and promote sustainability and community empowerment in health initiatives.
7. Analyze real-world case studies to demonstrate critical thinking and decision-making in the assessment, planning, implementation, and evaluation phases of community health nursing practice.
8. Differentiate between various community health nursing practice settings—including home health care, school health nursing, occupational health, and primary healthcare centers—and articulate the nurse's roles, responsibilities, and competencies in each.

R. I. Ashgar, *Community Health Nursing: Principles, Practices, and Perspectives*,
https://doi.org/10.1007/978-3-032-30791-0_6

9. Compare and contrast the unique challenges and opportunities associated with rural and urban health settings, with emphasis on accessibility, resource allocation, and population health equity.
10. Integrate principles of cultural respect, interprofessional collaboration, and ethical practice into community assessment and interventions across diverse community settings.

Understanding Community Dynamics

Community dynamics represent the complex interplay of various factors that influence the health and well-being of a community. Understanding these dynamics is crucial for community health nurses (CHNs), as it allows for the development of targeted interventions that address specific community needs. The social, economic, and environmental factors form the foundation upon which community health is built. Each community is unique, with its own set of challenges and resources, necessitating a tailored approach to health interventions [1].

Social factors include the population demographics, cultural norms, and social networks that define a community. These elements determine the community's health behaviors and attitudes towards health services. For instance, communities with strong social ties and networks may experience better health outcomes due to the support systems available. Conversely, communities with social fragmentation may face challenges such as increased rates of mental health issues and reduced access to healthcare services [2, 3].

Economic factors are equally pivotal in shaping community dynamics. The economic status of a community influences access to healthcare, nutrition, and education, all of which are critical determinants of health. Communities with limited economic resources often face barriers to accessing quality healthcare, leading to disparities in health outcomes. Economic stability allows for better healthcare infrastructure, availability of healthcare professionals, and access to medications and technologies [4].

Environmental factors encompass the physical surroundings of a community, including the quality of air, water, and housing. Environmental health hazards can have a profound impact on community health, contributing to conditions such as asthma, cardiovascular diseases, and other chronic illnesses. CHNs must assess environmental risks and advocate for policies that promote a healthy living environment [5].

Community dynamics are further influenced by political factors, including the governance structures and policies that dictate healthcare delivery. Effective leadership and governance can facilitate the implementation of health programs and ensure equitable access to healthcare services. Policies that prioritize community health can lead to improved health outcomes and reduced health disparities [6].

Understanding the interplay of these factors requires a comprehensive assessment of the community. This involves collecting data on health indicators, conducting surveys, and engaging with community members to identify their needs and priorities. CHNs play a pivotal role in this process, serving as liaisons between the community and healthcare providers. Interventions designed to improve community health must be evidence-based and culturally sensitive. This involves collaborating with community leaders and stakeholders to design programs that are acceptable and effective for the target population. CHNs must also evaluate the impact of these interventions, using data to refine and improve strategies over time.

In summary, understanding community dynamics is a foundational aspect of community health nursing. It enables nurses to develop interventions that are responsive to the unique needs of each community, ultimately leading to improved health outcomes and enhanced quality of life for community members. By considering the social, economic, environmental, and political factors that influence health, CHNs can effectively address health disparities and promote health equity.

Community Assessment

In the field of community health nursing, the assessment of a community is a critical process that involves the systematic collection, analysis, and dissemination of information about the health status of a community. This process is essential for identifying key health issues and needs, as well as for planning, implementing, and evaluating interventions aimed at improving community health outcomes [7]. Community assessment is a foundational step that informs the development of health policies and programs tailored to meet the unique needs of specific populations.

The process of community assessment typically begins with the identification of the community to be assessed. This involves defining the geographical boundaries of the community and understanding its demographic characteristics, such as age, gender, ethnicity, and socioeconomic status. It is crucial to engage community members and stakeholders in this process to ensure that the assessment is relevant and comprehensive. Engaging the community also helps to build trust and foster collaboration, which are vital for the successful implementation of health interventions [8].

Data collection is a core component of community assessment and can be achieved through various methods, including surveys, interviews, focus groups, and the review of existing public health data [9]. Quantitative data provide objective measures of health status, such as prevalence rates of diseases, mortality rates, and health service utilization. Qualitative data, on the other hand, offer insights into the lived experiences of community members, their perceptions of health issues, and the social and cultural factors that influence health behaviors. A mixed-methods approach, combining both quantitative and qualitative data, is often employed to provide a comprehensive understanding of the community's health status.

Once data are collected, the next step is data analysis, which involves organizing and interpreting the data to identify patterns, trends, and disparities in health outcomes. This analysis helps to pinpoint priority health issues that require immediate attention and resources. It is important to consider the social determinants of health, such as education, employment, housing, and access to healthcare, as these factors significantly impact the health and well being of communities [10].

The findings from the community assessment are then disseminated to stakeholders, including community members, health professionals, and policymakers. Effective communication of the results is crucial for garnering support and mobilizing resources for health interventions. The assessment results serve as a basis for developing evidence-based health policies and programs that address the identified health needs and priorities of the community.

In conclusion, community assessment is a dynamic and iterative process that requires ongoing collaboration and engagement with the community. It provides a critical foundation for community health nursing practice, enabling nurses to deliver culturally competent and effective care. By understanding the unique characteristics and needs of a community, health professionals can design interventions that are not only effective but also sustainable, ultimately leading to improved health outcomes and quality of life for community members.

Community Diagnosis

Community diagnosis is a fundamental outcome of analyzing assessment data in community health nursing. It involves the systematic identification of health-related issues, risks, and strengths within a specific population or geographic area [1, 3]. The diagnosis not only describes the current situation but also implies underlying causes or etiologies that contribute to the identified health status. This process focuses on the community as the client, emphasizing collective experiences and patterns rather than individual conditions. By examining these patterns, nurses gain insights into the social, environmental, and behavioral determinants that influence community wellness.

Unlike traditional nursing diagnoses that often focus on individual health deficits, CHNs adopt a broader perspective. They do not limit their analysis to problems alone; instead, they consider the community as an integrated system [2]. This holistic approach allows for the identification of both strengths and vulnerabilities. Nurses look for varied responses—both positive and negative—that affect the community's overall level of wellness. Through careful interpretation of assessment data, they infer both actual and potential problems and link them with contributing factors, crafting a comprehensive and context-specific diagnosis.

Each community diagnosis is composed of several key elements: the focus or population group, the inference or risk identified, the etiology or contributing factors, and the signs and symptoms that provide evidence of the problem. For instance, the senior residents of City A have the potential for achieving optimal functioning, which is inferred from their favorable health outcomes. This potential is related to multiple positive determinants such as access to exercise opportunities, healthcare services, and a healthy diet. These factors are manifested by observable indicators, including low mortality rates and a low prevalence of chronic conditions—evidence that supports the strength-based diagnosis.

Conversely, some community diagnoses highlight significant health risks. For example, the inhabitants of Town B in City A are at risk for illness and injury due to multiple hazardous conditions. These include exposure to pesticides, lack of safety knowledge, voluntary engagement in risky behaviors, insufficient family income to purchase safe equipment, and prolonged work hours leading to stress and fatigue. The manifestations of these risks are evident in the community's high prevalence of infectious diseases, frequent road injuries, and a low rate of vaccinations—factors that signify critical areas needing intervention.

Additionally, demographic-specific diagnoses reflect the unique challenges faced by particular groups. In Country A, middle-aged women are at increased risk for chronic conditions such as osteoporosis, breast cancer, and diabetes, largely attributable to unhealthy lifestyle practices. These include poor dietary habits, physical inactivity, and lack of engagement in preventive health behaviors. The diagnosis is supported by observable signs such as low rates of mammogram visits, infrequent breast self-examinations, and the absence of regular exercise routines. Addressing these risk factors is essential for improving health outcomes and enhancing preventive care strategies for this vulnerable population.

In conclusion, community diagnoses serve as a critical foundation for planning, implementing, and evaluating public health interventions. By identifying health strengths, risks, and contributing factors, nurses can tailor strategies that address the specific needs of the population while promoting overall wellness. This diagnostic process emphasizes the interconnectedness of individual and environmental factors, guiding practitioners to develop evidence-based, culturally sensitive, and sustainable health initiatives. As communities continue to face complex health challenges, accurate and comprehensive community diagnoses remain essential tools for achieving effective and equitable health outcomes.

Planning and Implementation

The process of planning and implementation in community health nursing involves a systematic approach to addressing the health needs of populations. This approach begins with a comprehensive assessment of the community to identify health issues and resources. The assessment phase is critical, as it provides the data needed to develop effective health strategies. Once the assessment is complete, the next step is to set priorities and goals. This involves analyzing the data to determine which health issues are most pressing and which can be realistically addressed with available resources. Setting priorities requires collaboration with community members and stakeholders to ensure that the selected goals are relevant and achievable. This collaborative approach not only enhances the relevance of the health interventions but also fosters community ownership and engagement [11].

The planning phase involves developing a detailed action plan that outlines the strategies and activities needed to achieve the set goals. This plan should include specific objectives, timelines, and the resources required for implementation. It is essential to consider the cultural, social, and economic factors that may influence the success of the health interventions. By tailoring strategies to the community's unique context, CHNs can enhance the effectiveness of their interventions [12].

Implementation is the phase where the planned activities are put into action. This requires careful coordination and management to ensure that the interventions are carried out as planned. During implementation, it is crucial to maintain flexibility and adaptability, as unforeseen challenges may arise. Continuous monitoring and evaluation are necessary to assess the progress of the interventions and to make necessary adjustments. This iterative process allows for the continuous improvement of health strategies and ensures that the interventions remain relevant and effective [12].

Throughout the planning and implementation process, communication plays a vital role. Effective communication ensures that all stakeholders are informed and engaged, which is essential for the success of the interventions. CHNs must also advocate for the necessary resources and support from local authorities and organizations. This advocacy is crucial for securing the funding and resources needed to sustain health interventions over the long term.

In conclusion, the planning and implementation of community health nursing interventions require a structured and collaborative approach. By engaging the community and working with stakeholders, CHNs can develop and implement strategies that effectively address the health needs of the population. This process not only improves health outcomes but also empowers communities to take an active role in their health and well-being.

Evaluation and Feedback

In the realm of community health nursing, the processes of evaluation and feedback serve as pivotal mechanisms that ensure the efficacy and continual improvement of health interventions [13]. These mechanisms are integral to the practice, allowing for the assessment of outcomes against established objectives and facilitating the refinement of strategies to better meet the needs of the community. Evaluation in community health nursing is a systematic process that involves the collection and analysis of data to determine the effectiveness of nursing interventions [1]. This process is not merely an endpoint but an ongoing cycle that informs future planning and decision-making. Evaluations are typically guided by specific criteria and standards that have been set in the planning phase of a program. These criteria might include health outcomes, changes in health behavior, or improvements in community health indicators. The evaluation process involves both quantitative and qualitative methods to provide a comprehensive picture of program impact.

Quantitative methods, such as surveys and statistical analysis, allow for the measurement of changes in health status or behavior, while qualitative methods, such as interviews and focus groups, provide insights into the experiences and perceptions of community members. This mixed-methods approach ensures a robust evaluation framework that captures both the tangible and intangible effects of health interventions.

Feedback, on the other hand, is the information derived from the evaluation process that is used to make informed decisions about program modifications. It serves as a communication tool between healthcare providers and the community, enabling the identification of areas that require improvement and the reinforcement of successful strategies. Feedback mechanisms should be timely, relevant, and specific to be effective. They should engage all stakeholders, including community members, healthcare professionals, and policymakers, to foster a collaborative approach to health improvement. The role of feedback in community health nursing extends beyond program adjustment; it is also a critical component of professional development. By reflecting on the outcomes of their interventions, nurses can identify skill gaps and areas for personal growth, thus enhancing their practice and the quality of care provided.

To maximize the impact of evaluation and feedback, it is essential to establish a culture of continuous improvement within community health organizations. This involves fostering an environment where learning from both successes and failures is encouraged and where feedback is valued as a tool for growth rather than criticism. Leadership plays a crucial role in this by promoting transparency, accountability, and a commitment to quality improvement.

Furthermore, the integration of technology into evaluation and feedback processes has transformed the way community health nursing operates. Digital tools for data collection and analysis have increased the efficiency and accuracy of evaluations, providing real-time insights that can be rapidly acted upon. These tools also facilitate the sharing of feedback across diverse teams and geographical locations, promoting a more coordinated and effective response to health challenges. In essence, evaluation and feedback are not mere adjuncts to community health nursing but are foundational elements that drive the advancement of the field [13]. By rigorously assessing interventions and incorporating feedback into practice, CHNs can ensure that their efforts are not only responsive to current health needs but are also adaptable to future challenges.

Case Studies

In the realm of community health nursing, case studies serve as a pivotal tool for exploring the multifaceted dynamics of health care delivery within communities. These narratives provide invaluable insights into the complex interactions between health professionals, patients, families, and the broader community context, illuminating the challenges and successes inherent in this field. The examination of case studies in community health nursing not only enhances understanding but also informs best practices and policy development.

One illustrative case study involves the management of chronic illness within a rural community. This scenario highlights the role of CHNs in coordinating care for individuals with limited access to healthcare facilities. The nurse acts as a liaison between the patient and various healthcare providers, ensuring continuity of care and adherence to treatment plans. This case underscores the importance of culturally competent care, as the nurse must navigate language barriers and differing health beliefs to effectively engage with the community.

Another case study focuses on health promotion and education in an urban setting, targeting school-age children and adolescents. This example illustrates the implementation of a school health program aimed at reducing the incidence of childhood obesity. CHNs collaborate with educators and parents to design and deliver educational sessions on nutrition and physical activity. The case study emphasizes the critical role of the nurse as an educator and advocate, working to empower young individuals to make informed health choices.

A third case study examines disaster management in a coastal community prone to hurricanes. Here, CHNs are integral to emergency preparedness and response efforts. They develop and implement community-wide education campaigns on disaster readiness, conduct drills, and coordinate with local emergency services. This case highlights the nurses' leadership and organizational skills, as well as their ability to foster resilience within the community.

The fourth case study explores the challenges of addressing environmental health concerns in an industrial town. CHNs collaborate with environmental scientists and policy makers to assess and mitigate the health impacts of industrial pollution. They conduct community health assessments, engage in public health advocacy, and facilitate community meetings to discuss environmental risks and health outcomes. This case underscores the importance of interdisciplinary collaboration in addressing complex public health issues.

Lastly, a case study on family violence intervention showcases the community health nurse's role in providing support and resources to affected families. Through home visits and partnerships with social services, nurses offer counseling, safety planning, and connections to community resources. This case highlights the nurse's role as a compassionate caregiver and a critical link in the support network for vulnerable populations.

These case studies collectively demonstrate the diverse roles of CHNs and the impact they have on improving health outcomes. Through their work, they address a wide range of health issues, from chronic disease management to disaster preparedness, all while advocating for policy changes that promote health equity. The lessons learned from these case studies are invaluable for shaping the future of community health nursing, guiding both practice and policy to better serve communities.

Settings for Community Health Nursing

Home Health Care

Home health care represents a pivotal component of community health nursing, focusing on delivering personalized health services directly to individuals in their residences. This approach not only enhances the accessibility of healthcare but also fosters an environment conducive to recovery and well-being by allowing patients to remain in familiar surroundings [14]. The integration of home health care into community health nursing underscores the commitment to holistic and patient-centered care, emphasizing the importance of addressing the diverse needs of individuals across various settings [1, 3, 10].

The provision of home health care involves a multidisciplinary team of healthcare professionals, including nurses, physicians, therapists, and social workers, who collaborate to develop and implement comprehensive care plans tailored to the unique needs of each patient. This collaborative framework ensures that patients receive a continuum of care that addresses their medical, psychological, and social needs, thereby promoting optimal health outcomes.

One of the primary objectives of home health care is to reduce the need for hospitalization and long-term institutional care, which can be both costly and disruptive to patients' lives [3]. By providing timely and efficient healthcare services at home, community health nurses (CHNs) play a crucial role in preventing complications, managing chronic conditions, and facilitating recovery from acute illnesses or surgeries. This proactive approach not only enhances the quality of life for patients but also alleviates the burden on healthcare systems by decreasing the demand for inpatient services.

Home health care also emphasizes the importance of patient and family education, empowering individuals to take an active role in managing their health [3]. CHNs serve as educators and advocates, providing patients and their families with the knowledge and skills necessary to make informed decisions about their care. This educational component is vital in promoting self-management, adherence to treatment plans, and the adoption of healthy lifestyle behaviors, all of which contribute to improved health outcomes and reduced healthcare costs.

Moreover, home health care addresses the social determinants of health by recognizing the impact of environmental, economic, and social factors on individuals' well-being. By delivering care in the home setting, CHNs can identify and address potential barriers to health, such as inadequate housing, lack of social support, or limited access to resources [10]. This comprehensive approach enhances the ability of healthcare providers to offer targeted interventions that address the root causes of health disparities and promote health equity within communities.

In the context of an aging population and an increasing prevalence of chronic diseases, home health care is poised to play an increasingly vital role in the healthcare landscape [15]. As community health nursing continues to evolve, the integration of technology, such as telehealth and remote monitoring, is expanding the reach and effectiveness of home healthcare services. These advancements enable healthcare providers to deliver high-quality care to patients in remote or underserved areas, further enhancing the accessibility and efficiency of healthcare delivery.

In summary, home health care is an essential component of community health nursing that offers numerous benefits for patients, healthcare providers, and the broader healthcare system. By delivering patient-centered, comprehensive, and accessible care in the home setting, CHNs are at the forefront of efforts to improve health outcomes, reduce healthcare costs, and promote health equity. As the demand for home health care continues to grow, ongoing innovation and collaboration among healthcare professionals will be crucial in meeting the evolving needs of patients and communities.

Scope of Home Health Care

Home health care refers to a wide range of clinical and supportive services provided to individuals in their homes. Services may include nursing care, physical therapy, occupational therapy, speech therapy, medication management, wound care, and patient education.

The Saudi Context

The concept of home health care, where professional nursing care is brought directly into the patient's residence, represents a significant evolution in healthcare delivery globally. In the Kingdom of Saudi Arabia, driven by rapid modernization, an aging population, and a growing emphasis on family-centric care, home health nursing has emerged as a vital component of the healthcare landscape. As nurses working within this context, their role extends beyond the hospital walls into the very heart of families' homes, offering care, support, and education in a setting deeply rooted in cultural values [16].

Understanding home health care in Saudi Arabia necessitates a brief glance at the societal backdrop. The family, particularly the extended family, remains the cornerstone of social and economic life. Respect for elders and deep-seated beliefs about health and illness shape healthcare preferences and practices. Traditionally, care for the sick and elderly was predominantly provided by family members, often women within the household. However, alongside rapid urbanization, economic development, and increased life expectancy, there is a growing demand for professional medical services, including those delivered at home.

This shift is influenced by factors such as:

1. **Aging Population:** Like many developed nations, Saudi Arabia is experiencing population aging, leading to a higher prevalence of chronic illnesses requiring ongoing management.
2. **Chronic Disease Burden:** Non-communicable diseases, such as diabetes, hypertension, and heart disease, are major health concerns. Home health care plays a crucial role in managing these conditions through regular monitoring, medication management, and patient education.
3. **Technological Advancement:** Improved communication infrastructure and the integration of telehealth are making home-based care more feasible and efficient.
4. **Economic Considerations:** While still developing, the private sector is increasingly investing in home health services, recognizing the potential cost-effectiveness compared to prolonged hospital stays, especially for complex cases.
5. **Desire for Comfort:** Many patients and their families prefer to receive care in the familiar and comforting environment of their homes, surrounded by family and familiar objects.

Goals of Home Health Care in Saudi Arabia

1. Promote the independence and dignity of patients.
2. Reduce unnecessary hospital admissions and readmissions.
3. Facilitate post-hospital discharge care.
4. Improve patient outcomes and satisfaction.
5. Provide culturally appropriate and family-oriented care.

The Role of the Community Health Nurse in Home Health Care

In this evolving landscape, nurses assume a multifaceted role. They are not merely providers of medical care; they are cultural brokers, educators, assessors, supporters, and advocates.

- **Assessment:** The initial step involves a comprehensive assessment within the home environment. This goes beyond the patient's physical health. Nurses evaluate the home setting for safety (e.g., navigating stairs, potential hazards), accessibility, available support systems (family members), and the patient's functional abilities. Understanding the family's dynamics, roles, and cultural beliefs is paramount. For instance, assessing the health needs of a female patient requires careful consideration of gender norms and the need for female nurses.
- **Care Planning:** Based on the assessment, nurses collaboratively develop a care plan with the patient (where appropriate), their family, and the referring physician. This plan outlines specific nursing interventions, education goals, medication schedules, and follow-up requirements. It must be flexible, adapting to the unique circumstances of each home and family.
- **Direct Patient Care:** This includes a wide range of services: administering medications, performing wound care, monitoring vital signs, assisting with activities of daily living (ADLs) such as bathing and dressing (respecting cultural norms), providing pain management, and interpreting diagnostic tests.
- **Patient and Family Education:** A significant portion of their role involves educating patients and their families. This extends beyond technical medical information. Nurses educate patients and their families about chronic disease self-management (e.g., insulin administration for diabetes, blood pressure monitoring, dietary modifications according to cultural preferences and health needs). They also empower them to recognize signs of deterioration and know when to seek further help.
- **Advocacy and Resource Navigation:** Nurses act as advocates for their patients, ensuring their needs and concerns are heard by the healthcare team. They also help families navigate the complex healthcare system, connecting them with necessary resources, community services, and support groups.
- **Documentation and Coordination:** Meticulous documentation of care provided, patient progress, and communication with other healthcare providers is essential. They often serve as a crucial link between the hospital, clinics, and the patient's home, ensuring continuity of care.

Challenges and Opportunities

Practicing home health care in Saudi Arabia is rewarding but not without its challenges [17].

- **Logistical Hurdles:** Navigating cities, which can have challenging traffic, requires careful planning. Accessing certain neighborhoods, especially in smaller towns or

rural areas, might be limited. Weather conditions, particularly extreme heat in the summer, can impact scheduling and patient comfort.
- **Cultural Barriers:** While cultural respect is paramount, navigating subtle nuances and ensuring all family members are comfortable with the care provided can be complex. Balancing the patient's needs with strong family desires requires diplomacy and patience.
- **Workforce Shortages**: One of the most pressing challenges facing the home health care is the limited number of trained CHNs with home care experience

However, these challenges are counterbalanced by significant opportunities. The growing demand for home health services offers a unique platform for nurses to make a meaningful impact. It allows for direct involvement in preventive care and health promotion, fostering a public health approach within communities. The increasing integration of technology presents exciting possibilities for remote monitoring and enhanced communication. Most importantly, it offers the chance to build deep, personal connections with patients and families, providing care that is both professional and deeply human.

School Health Nursing

School health nursing is a specialized field of community health nursing that focuses on delivering healthcare services within the school setting. The integration of health services within the educational environment is pivotal in fostering a holistic approach to child and adolescent health [18]. School health nursing encompasses a broad spectrum of activities and programs designed to enhance the physical, mental, and social well-being of students. These services operate within a framework that acknowledges the unique needs of school-aged children and adolescents, recognizing the school setting as a critical platform for health promotion and disease prevention [19, 20]. School health services are essential in ensuring that students achieve optimal health, which is foundational for effective learning and academic success [1].

The core components of school health nursing include health screenings, immunizations, management of chronic conditions, emergency care, and health education. Health screenings are crucial for the early detection of health issues that may impede a student's ability to learn. Regular screenings for vision, hearing, and dental health, as well as assessments for growth and development, are standard practices in school health services. Immunization programs within schools play a significant role in controlling the spread of infectious diseases. Schools serve as an accessible venue for delivering vaccinations, ensuring high coverage rates among students. This not only protects individual students but also contributes to herd immunity, safeguarding the broader community.

Moreover, the management of chronic conditions, such as asthma and diabetes, is a vital component of school health services. School nurses and health personnel are trained to provide care and support for students with chronic health issues, allowing them to participate fully in school activities without disruption. Emergency care is another critical aspect of school health services. Schools must be equipped to respond promptly and effectively to health emergencies, minimizing the risk of severe outcomes. This involves having trained personnel, emergency protocols, and necessary medical supplies readily available. Furthermore, health education is an integral part of school health services, aiming to equip students with the knowledge and skills needed to make informed health decisions. This includes education on nutrition, physical activity, mental health, substance abuse prevention, and sexual health.

The role of school health nursing extends beyond addressing immediate health needs. These services are instrumental in promoting a culture of health within the school community, influencing students' health behaviors and attitudes. Collaboration between health professionals, educators, and parents is essential to create a supportive environment that prioritizes student health and well-being. School health nursing also plays a critical role in addressing health disparities, ensuring that all students, regardless of socioeconomic status, have access to necessary health resources and support.

In conclusion, school health nursing is a fundamental component of community health nursing, bridging the gap between healthcare and education. By addressing the health needs of students, these services contribute significantly to their overall development and success. The effective implementation of school health services requires a coordinated approach that involves multi-disciplinary collaboration, adequate resources, and policy support. Through these efforts, school health services can fulfill their potential in promoting the health and academic achievement of students, ultimately contributing to the well-being of the entire community.

The Saudi Context

In Saudi Arabia, with more than 30% of the population under 18 years old, school health nursing plays a crucial role in supporting child and adolescent well-being [21]. The responsibility for school health services is jointly managed by the Ministry of Health (MOH) and the Ministry of Education, which work together to implement health programs, train personnel, and lead nationwide health initiatives targeting students' health [22]. The MOH has launched the «Healthy Schools» Program to improve the health of students in accordance with the global standards, policies, and procedures of the World Health Organization (WHO) [23]. The National Healthy School Program, which aligns with the goals of Saudi Vision 2030, aims to:

- Acquire knowledge, develop skills, and improve health habits of school community members.
- Activate and motivate students to participate effectively in health promotion activities at schools.
- Create a healthy and safe school environment.
- Strengthen ties between different schools.
- Promote the health of school staff.
- Strengthen ties and cooperation between the school community and society.

The Role and Responsibilities of the School Health Nurse

1. **Health Promoters:** They develop and implement health education programs covering topics such as personal hygiene, nutrition, physical activity, substance abuse prevention, mental health awareness, and safety practices (road safety, disaster preparedness).
2. **Disease Detectors and Managers:** They conduct routine health screenings (vision, hearing, dental, growth measurements), manage chronic conditions among students (e.g., administering insulin, monitoring blood glucose levels, managing asthma), and respond to acute health episodes. They play a crucial role in early detection and referral for suspected health issues.
3. **Immunization Coordinators:** They ensure students are in compliance with national immunization requirements, manage vaccination campaigns within the school, and maintain accurate immunization records.
4. **Health Advocates:** They advocate for the health needs of students within the school system, working with teachers, administrators, and parents to create a supportive and healthy school environment. This includes advocating for policies that promote healthy nutrition (e.g., vending machine regulations), adequate physical activity time, and mental health support services.
5. **Communicators:** They serve as a vital link between the school, students, families, and the broader healthcare system. They communicate with parents about health concerns or required treatments, provide health advice, and coordinate referrals to primary healthcare clinics or specialists when needed. Maintaining clear and respectful communication, considering cultural norms, is essential.
6. **Safety Officers:** They contribute to ensuring a safe school environment by assessing potential hazards, implementing safety protocols, and training staff and students on emergency procedures.

Challenges and Opportunities

Challenges:

1. **Workforce Shortages:** There is a shortage of nurses with specialized training in school health. Many schools do not have full-time nurses, particularly in rural or underserved areas.
2. **Resource Limitations:** Some schools, particularly in less developed areas or smaller institutions, may lack adequate facilities, equipment, or essential supplies for comprehensive health services.
3. **Scope of Practice:** There is a lack of unified national policies or guidelines regarding the scope of practice, job descriptions, and performance standards for school nurses.
4. **Workload:** School nurses often have heavy caseloads and multiple responsibilities, demanding versatility and strong organizational skills.

Opportunities:

1. **Visibility and Impact:** School nurses have daily, consistent contact with a large number of students, offering unparalleled opportunities to impact health behaviors and outcomes on a large scale.
2. **Preventive Focus:** The school setting is ideal for implementing preventive health measures, potentially reducing illness and healthcare costs in the long run.
3. **Partnerships:** There is growing potential for collaboration between school nurses, healthcare providers, public health agencies, and community organizations to develop comprehensive school health programs.
4. **Evolving Role:** As the importance of holistic health (including mental and social well-being) gains recognition, the role of school nurses is expanding to encompass these areas, offering exciting professional development opportunities.

Occupational Health

Occupational health is a critical component of community health nursing, focusing on the identification and management of health and safety risks in the workplace. This subchapter delves into the various factors that contribute to occupational health, including physical, chemical, biological, ergonomic, and psychosocial hazards. The role of CHNs in occupational health involves not only the prevention and management of work-related illnesses and injuries but also the promotion of health and well-being among workers.

Physical hazards in the workplace can include noise, vibration, radiation, and extreme temperatures. These factors can have detrimental effects on workers' health, leading to conditions such as hearing loss, musculoskeletal disorders, and heat-related illnesses. CHNs play a vital role in assessing these risks and implementing strategies to mitigate their impact, such as advocating for the use of personal protective equipment and promoting workplace safety training [10].

Chemical hazards are another significant concern in occupational health. Exposure to hazardous substances, such as solvents, pesticides, and heavy metals, can lead to acute or chronic health issues, including respiratory problems, skin conditions, and even cancer. CHNs are instrumental in educating workers about the safe handling and disposal of chemicals, as well as monitoring workplaces for compliance with safety regulations [10].

Biological hazards, including bacteria, viruses, and fungi, pose a risk to workers in various sectors, particularly healthcare and agriculture. These hazards can lead to infectious diseases, which can spread rapidly if not properly managed. CHNs are crucial in identifying potential biological risks, implementing infection control measures, and providing immunizations to at-risk populations [3].

Ergonomic hazards arise from poor workplace design and can result in musculoskeletal injuries, such as carpal tunnel syndrome and back pain. CHNs assess workstations and recommend modifications to improve ergonomics, thereby reducing the incidence of these injuries. They also educate workers on proper body mechanics and the importance of taking regular breaks to prevent strain [3].

Psychosocial hazards in the workplace, such as stress, harassment, and job insecurity, can have profound effects on mental health. These factors can lead to anxiety, depression, and burnout, impacting both individual workers and overall workplace productivity. CHNs support workers by providing counseling services, facilitating stress management programs, and advocating for policies that promote a positive work environment [3].

In summary, occupational health is an integral part of community health nursing, addressing the diverse health risks present in work environments. Through comprehensive risk assessment, education, and intervention, CHNs play a pivotal role in safeguarding the health and well-being of workers. Their efforts not only reduce the incidence of work-related illnesses and injuries but also contribute to healthier, more productive communities.

The Saudi Context

The workplace is a cornerstone of any modern economy, driving productivity, innovation, and national development. In the rapidly evolving landscape of Saudi Arabia, characterized by ambitious economic diversification initiatives such as Vision 2030, the workforce is expanding and encountering new challenges and opportunities [24]. Within this context, ensuring the health and safety of employees is paramount not only for ethical reasons and employee well-being but also for maintaining operational efficiency and national competitiveness. Occupational health nursing plays a critical role in this sphere, acting as a sentinel for worker health, a promoter of safe practices, and an advocate for a healthy work environment.

The Role and Responsibilities of the Occupational Health Nurse

Occupational health nurses work within various settings—companies' internal health departments, dedicated occupational health clinics, or public health institutions supporting industries. Their role is proactive, preventative, and often multidimensional. Key responsibilities include:

- **Health Surveillance:** Conducting baseline health assessments for new employees and periodic monitoring for existing staff to identify early signs of work-related illness or exposure effects. This might involve respiratory function tests, blood pressure monitoring, or specific chemical exposure screening, depending on the industry.
- **Risk Assessment and Management:** Collaborating with engineers, safety officers, and management to identify potential hazards in the workplace (e.g., chemical exposures, noise levels, ergonomic risks, fire hazards, psychosocial risks such as

burnout or violence). They contribute to developing and implementing control measures to minimize these risks, ensuring compliance with local regulations.

- **Health Education and Promotion:** Implementing educational programs for employees on a wide range of topics, including safe use of equipment, proper manual handling techniques, importance of personal protective equipment (PPE), hazard communication, substance abuse prevention, stress management, and reproductive health concerns specific to the workplace (e.g., heat stress, chemical exposure during pregnancy).
- **Emergency Preparedness and Response:** Developing and conducting drills for workplace emergencies (e.g., fires, chemical spills, medical emergencies). They are often the first responders, ensuring immediate care is provided and coordinating with emergency services.
- **Workplace Injury and Illness Management:** Managing work-related injuries and illnesses, providing initial care, coordinating referrals to specialists, facilitating return-to-work processes, and investigating incidents to prevent recurrence.
- **Promoting a Positive Health Culture:** Acting as a resource person for employees' health concerns, fostering open communication about safety and health, and promoting a culture where employee well-being is prioritized by management.

Challenges and Opportunities

Challenges:

1. **Resource Allocation:** Securing adequate funding, staffing, and necessary equipment within some organizations, particularly smaller or less established ones.
2. **Regulatory Clarity and Enforcement:** Navigating evolving regulations and ensuring consistent enforcement across all sectors and regions.
3. **Silence on Reporting:** Overcoming barriers to reporting health concerns or safety hazards, which can be influenced by fear of retribution, cultural norms, or lack of awareness of rights.
4. **Worker Mobility:** Addressing health and safety issues for workers in precarious or temporary employment, or those moving between different jobs frequently.

Opportunities:

1. **Growing Recognition:** Increasing awareness and buy-in from employers regarding the importance of occupational health for productivity, employee morale, and reputation.
2. **National Development Needs:** The ongoing economic diversification creates a need for skilled occupational health professionals to support new and expanding industries.
3. **Technology Integration:** Leveraging technology for remote monitoring, digital health education platforms, and improved incident reporting systems.

4. **Expanding Role:** The evolving focus on holistic health, including mental well-being and work-life balance, offers an expanding scope for nurses to contribute.

Primary Healthcare Centers

Primary healthcare centers (PHCs) serve as a cornerstone in the community health landscape, offering essential services that address a wide range of health needs. These centers are strategically positioned to provide accessible and affordable healthcare to diverse populations, particularly underserved communities. They operate with a focus on preventive care, chronic disease management, and health education, which are crucial components in reducing healthcare disparities and promoting overall community well-being [25].

Within PHCs, a multidisciplinary team of healthcare professionals collaborates to deliver comprehensive services. This team typically includes physicians, nurses, social workers, and health educators, each playing a vital role in patient care. Nurses, in particular, are pivotal in these settings due to their expertise in community health nursing. They engage in direct patient care, conduct health assessments, and develop care plans tailored to the specific needs of the community. By doing so, they help bridge the gap between patients and the healthcare system, ensuring that individuals receive the necessary care and support.

PHCs also emphasize the importance of preventive care services, which are designed to avert the onset of diseases and health conditions. These services include immunizations, screenings for various health conditions such as hypertension and diabetes, and counseling on lifestyle modifications. By focusing on prevention, PHCs aim to reduce the incidence of diseases, thereby decreasing the overall burden on the healthcare system and improving quality of life [26].

In addition to preventive services, PHCs play a crucial role in managing chronic diseases. Chronic conditions such as diabetes, heart disease, and asthma require ongoing monitoring and management to prevent complications. PHCs provide regular check-ups, medication management, and education on self-care practices. This continuous support is essential for patients to maintain their health and prevent hospitalizations [27].

Health education is another critical component of the services offered by PHCs. Educating the community about health risks, healthy behaviors, and available resources empowers individuals to make informed decisions about their health. PHCs often conduct workshops, seminars, and outreach programs that address topics such as nutrition, physical activity, mental health, and substance abuse prevention. By increasing health literacy, these clinics contribute to the development of healthier communities [25, 26].

Moreover, PHCs are instrumental in addressing public health emergencies and outbreaks. During such events, they serve as vital points for disseminating information, administering vaccines, and providing treatment to affected individuals. Their ability to mobilize resources quickly and efficiently makes them indispensable in safeguarding community health during crises [25, 26].

Overall, PHCs are integral to the healthcare infrastructure, providing essential services that enhance the health and well-being of communities. Through their focus on prevention, chronic disease management, and health education, they not only improve individual health outcomes but also contribute to the reduction of healthcare costs. As the healthcare landscape continues to evolve, PHCs will remain a vital resource for communities, adapting to meet emerging health challenges and ensuring that all individuals have access to quality care.

The Saudi Context

PHCs are vital institutions in the Saudi healthcare system, playing a foundational role in disease prevention, health promotion, and the delivery of essential community-based services. These clinics support the broader goals of the Saudi Vision 2030 by focusing on population health, early detection, and reducing the burden on hospitals [26]. CHNs are central to the function and success of these clinics, acting as front-line providers who assess, educate, treat, and empower individuals and families within their communities.

PHCs are government-funded or community-based facilities that deliver primary and preventive health services. Unlike hospitals, which focus on curative and acute care, PHCs emphasize:

- Health education and awareness
- Immunization and infectious disease control
- Maternal and child health services
- Chronic disease screening and management
- Environmental health
- Nutritional counseling
- Community outreach and epidemiological surveillance

These centers are often embedded in neighborhoods and rural areas, ensuring healthcare access for all segments of the population, especially underserved or vulnerable groups.

The Role of Community Health Nurses in PHCs

Community health nurses are the backbone of PHCs. Their diverse responsibilities include:

1. Health Assessment and Primary Care Services
CHNs conduct initial assessments, vital signs monitoring, and basic physical examinations for clients visiting the PHCs. They help identify potential health risks early and provide guidance or referrals to specialized care. In many cases, they serve as the first point of contact in the health system, especially in rural and underserved areas where physicians may be limited.

2. Health Promotion and Education

Education is a major pillar of the community health nurse's role. Nurses provide individualized and group health education tailored to the cultural and religious context of the community. Health promotion activities are designed to empower individuals to make informed decisions about their health.

3. Immunization and Communicable Disease Control

CHNs play a central role in national immunization programs. They administer vaccines according to MOH schedules and ensure that coverage is maintained within their communities.

- Administer childhood and adult vaccinations
- Maintain immunization records and monitor vaccine coverage rates
- Identify and respond to outbreaks of communicable diseases (e.g., influenza, measles, COVID-19)
- Implement infection control measures within clinic settings

4. Maternal and Child Health Services

One of the most important roles of CHNs in public health clinics is supporting maternal, neonatal, and child health (MNCH).

- Provide prenatal and postnatal counseling and assessments
- Monitor child growth and development through well-baby clinics
- Promote exclusive breastfeeding and proper infant nutrition
- Educate mothers about child spacing and family planning

5. Management of Chronic and Non-Communicable Diseases (NCDs)

CHNs are deeply involved in the early detection and ongoing management of chronic conditions, which are prevalent in Saudi Arabia, including diabetes, hypertension, and obesity.

- Conduct risk assessments and screenings for NCDs
- Monitor treatment adherence and patient outcomes
- Counsel patients on medication management, diet, and physical activity
- Coordinate with physicians to adjust treatment plans as needed

6. Mental Health Support and Counseling

With the growing recognition of mental health as a public health priority, CHNs are increasingly involved in early identification and basic support for clients experiencing mental distress.

- Identify early signs of anxiety, depression, or emotional distress
- Offer initial counseling or listening support
- Refer patients to specialized mental health services when needed
- Provide psychoeducation to reduce stigma around mental health

7. Home Visits and Community Outreach

CHNs may conduct home visits, particularly for elderly patients, individuals with disabilities, and mothers with newborns. These visits are especially important in rural areas where access to health facilities may be limited.

- Assess living conditions and home environments for health hazards
- Provide follow-up care after hospitalization
- Educate families on hygiene, nutrition, and home-based care practices
- Connect families to social services and resources

8. Health Surveillance and Data Collection

CHNs support public health planning and policymaking by collecting, documenting, and reporting health data at the local level.

- Maintain patient records and health statistics
- Monitor trends in disease incidence and health behaviors
- Report notifiable diseases to health authorities
- Participate in research or pilot programs for public health improvement

9. Emergency Response and Crisis Management

During public health emergencies (e.g., disease outbreaks, natural disasters, or mass gatherings such as Hajj), CHNs serve as vital responders.

- Participate in vaccination campaigns or emergency preparedness drills
- Deliver care and health education in mobile clinics or temporary shelters
- Educate the public about emergency protocols and hygiene during crises

10. Collaboration and Interdisciplinary Coordination

CHNs in PHCs work closely with a wide range of healthcare providers, educators, religious leaders, and social service agencies to address the broader determinants of health.

- Coordinate with primary care physicians, nutritionists, and social workers
- Advocate for patients and assist them in navigating healthcare systems
- Participate in inter-ministerial projects involving education, housing, or environmental safety

Challenges Facing PHCs in Saudi Arabia

Despite their importance, PHCs face several systemic and operational challenges [28]:

1. **Staffing Shortages:** There remains a shortage of trained Saudi CHNs and other allied health professionals, especially in rural regions.
2. **Public Awareness and Utilization:** Many citizens prefer hospitals for even minor issues, due to a lack of awareness about PHCs services or perceptions of lower quality.
3. **Coordination with Other Sectors:** Linkages between clinics, schools, municipalities, and social services are limited, reducing the impact of cross-sectoral health initiatives.

Vision 2030 and the Future of PHCs

Saudi Arabia's Vision 2030 is a comprehensive national reform plan designed to diversify the economy, modernize public services, and enhance the quality of life for all citizens and residents [29]. Healthcare transformation is one of the central pillars of this vision, and PHCs are poised to play a leading role in achieving its health-related objectives. These centers are the front line of community-based, preventive, and promotive care, and their future is closely tied to the realization of Vision 2030 goals [29].

1. Shift from Curative to Preventive Care

One of the primary objectives of Vision 2030's Health Sector Transformation Program is to reduce the Kingdom's reliance on hospital-based, curative services and focus more on preventive, primary, and community health care [26]. PHCs are expected to:

- Provide early screening and detection of chronic illnesses (e.g., diabetes, hypertension, obesity)
- Promote healthy lifestyles through education, counseling, and public campaigns
- Offer comprehensive immunization services for children and adults
- Support mental health awareness and early intervention
- Implement tobacco cessation and nutrition programs

This shift helps reduce healthcare costs and ensures better long-term health outcomes.

2. Enhancing Accessibility and Equity

Vision 2030 emphasizes equitable access to quality healthcare across all regions of the Kingdom, including underserved and remote communities [25]. PHCs are being upgraded and expanded to fulfill this vision by:

- Expanding services in rural areas where healthcare infrastructure is limited
- Integrating mobile health units and telehealth services to reach remote populations
- Establishing new PHCs with advanced diagnostic tools and more specialized services

This ensures that all individuals, regardless of geography or socioeconomic status, have access to essential health services.

3. Improving Quality and Efficiency of Care

Vision 2030 calls for significant improvements in healthcare quality, efficiency, and patient satisfaction [25]. To meet these goals, PHCs are undergoing reforms such as:

- **Digital Transformation**: Introduction of electronic medical records, appointment systems, and data-sharing platforms through tools such as the Sehhaty app and Mawid system.
- **Accreditation and Standardization:** PHCs are increasingly required to meet national standards for service delivery, safety, and infection control, supported

by the Saudi Central Board for Accreditation of Healthcare Institutions (CBAHI).

Training and Capacity Building: Investments in the education and continuing development of healthcare professionals to improve competencies in public health practice.

4. Integration of PHCs into a Unified Health System

Vision 2030 envisions a coordinated, integrated healthcare system where primary, secondary, and tertiary care facilities work together seamlessly. Public health clinics are being restructured to serve as the entry point into the healthcare system, with better referral and feedback mechanisms:

- Coordinating care with hospitals and specialist centers
- Managing patients with chronic diseases through a family medicine model
- Offering continuity of care and case management through a patient-centered approach

5. Public–Private Partnerships (PPP)

Vision 2030 encourages the privatization and diversification of healthcare services, including the development of public–private partnerships (PPPs) [30]. Public health clinics may be managed by private operators under government regulation, allowing:

- Improved efficiency and innovation in service delivery
- Increased investment in infrastructure and technologies
- Expansion of specialized services such as dental care, mental health counseling, and laboratory testing

This model aims to reduce the financial burden on the government while enhancing service options for the population.

6. Focus on Health Literacy and Community Engagement

An empowered population is a key theme in Vision 2030. Public health clinics are central to promoting health literacy and engaging communities through:

- Grassroots health education initiatives
- Collaboration with schools, mosques, and community centers
- Training community health volunteers and peer educators
- Delivering culturally appropriate health messages that resonate with local values and traditions

These efforts aim to cultivate a culture of prevention, responsibility, and self-care.

7. Data-Driven Public Health and Research

Another focus of Vision 2030 is building a data-driven healthcare system [31]. PHCs are being positioned as essential sources of public health surveillance data, including:

- Disease trends and outbreaks

- Health behavior indicators
- Population health outcomes

These data support evidence-based policymaking and help the government track progress toward national health goals. It also strengthens Saudi Arabia's capacity to respond to emergencies, such as epidemics and environmental health crises.

Rural and Urban Settings

In the realm of community health nursing, the differentiation between rural and urban settings presents distinct challenges and opportunities for healthcare providers. These settings are defined by unique demographic, socioeconomic, and environmental characteristics that influence health outcomes and access to care.

Rural areas are often characterized by sparse populations, limited healthcare infrastructure, and significant distances between healthcare facilities. This geographical isolation can lead to difficulties in accessing timely medical care, which are compounded by a shortage of healthcare professionals willing to practice in these areas. Additionally, rural populations tend to have higher rates of chronic diseases, such as hypertension and diabetes, partly due to lifestyle factors and limited access to preventive services. The socioeconomic status in rural settings often reflects lower income levels and higher rates of unemployment, which can further restrict access to necessary healthcare services [32].

In contrast, urban settings, while having more readily available healthcare facilities and professionals, face their own set of challenges. Urban areas are typically densely populated, which can lead to overcrowding in healthcare facilities and longer wait times for patients. The fast-paced lifestyle in urban settings, along with higher levels of pollution and stress, contributes to a different spectrum of health issues, including mental health disorders and respiratory illnesses. Despite the proximity of healthcare services, disparities in access still exist, particularly for marginalized communities that may face financial barriers or discrimination within the healthcare system [32].

The role of CHNs in these settings is pivotal. In rural areas, nurses often serve as primary healthcare providers, delivering a wide range of services from acute care to health education and disease prevention. They are essential in building trust within the community and tailoring health interventions to meet the specific needs of the population. This requires nurses to be adaptable and resourceful, often working with limited resources and in collaboration with local organizations to maximize health outcomes. In urban environments, CHNs play a crucial role in navigating the complex healthcare landscape. They work to bridge gaps in care by advocating for underserved populations and coordinating care across various services. Their efforts in health promotion and disease prevention are vital in managing the public health concerns that arise from urban living conditions.

Furthermore, the integration of technology in both rural and urban settings enhances the ability of CHNs to deliver care. Telehealth services have become increasingly important, particularly in rural areas, by providing remote consultations and reducing the need for travel. In urban settings, electronic health records and mobile health applications facilitate better management of patient care and health education. Ultimately, the effectiveness of CHNs in rural and urban settings hinges on the ability to understand and respond to the specific health needs of each community. By leveraging local resources, fostering community partnerships, and employing innovative healthcare delivery methods, CHNs can significantly improve health outcomes and reduce disparities across these diverse environments.

References

1. Stanhope M, Lancaster J. Public health nursing: population-centered health care in the community. 11th ed. Elsevier; 2024.
2. Anderson ET, McFarlane J. Community as partner: theory and practice in nursing. 8th ed. Lippincott Williams & Wilkins; 2018.
3. Nies MA, McEwen M. Community/public health nursing: promoting the health of populations. 8th ed. Elsevier; 2023.
4. Cobigo V, Martin L, Rawad M. Understanding community. Can J Disabil Stud. 2016;5(4):181. https://doi.org/10.15353/cjds.v5i4.318.
5. Ravaghi H, Guisset AL, Elfeky S, Nasir N, Khani S, Ahmadnezhad E, et al. A scoping review of community health needs and assets assessment: concepts, rationale, tools and uses. BMC Health Serv Res. 2023;23(1):44. https://doi.org/10.1186/s12913-022-08983-3.
6. Harkness G. Community and public health nursing: evidence for practice. Wolters Kluwer; 2016.
7. Pazzaglia C, Camedda C, Ugenti NV, Trentin A, Scalorbi S, Longobucco Y. Community health assessment tools adoptable in nursing practice: a scoping review. Int J Environ Res Public Health. 2023;20(3):1667. https://doi.org/10.3390/ijerph20031667.
8. Silberberg M, Cook J, Drescher C, McCloskey D. Principles of community engagement. 2nd ed. NIH Publication No. 11-7782. National Institutes of Health; 2011.
9. Goodman RA, Bunnell R, Posner SF. What is "community health"? Examining the meaning of an evolving field in public health. Prev Med. 2014;67(Suppl 1):S58–61. https://doi.org/10.1016/j.ypmed.2014.07.028.
10. Seabert T, McKenzie J, Pinger R. An introduction to community and public health. 10th ed. Jones & Bartlett Learning; 2021.
11. Barry MM, Clarke AM, Petersen I, Jenkins R. Implementing mental health promotion. Springer; 2019.
12. Nickel S, von dem Knesebeck O. Effectiveness of community-based health promotion interventions in urban areas: a systematic review. J Community Health. 2020;45(2):419–34. https://doi.org/10.1007/s10900-019-00733-7.
13. Adams J, Neville S. Program evaluation for health professionals: what it is, what it isn't and how to do it. Int J Qual Methods. 2020;19:1609406920964345. https://doi.org/10.1177/1609406920964345.
14. Al-Surimi K, Al-Harbi I, El-Metwally A, Badri M. Quality of life among home healthcare patients in Saudi Arabia: household-based survey. Health Qual Life Outcomes. 2019;17(1):21. https://doi.org/10.1186/s12955-019-1095-z.
15. Alabbasi KH, Kruger E, Tennant M. Long term implications of home healthcare management on mortality in older adults with functional difficulties in the Saudi community. Geriatrics (Basel). 2021;6(4):115. https://doi.org/10.3390/geriatrics6040115.
16. Ministry of Health (Saudi Arabia). Home health care services [Internet]. 2024 [cited 2026 Feb 17]. Available from: https://www.moh.gov.sa/en/awarenessplateform/Patientsrights/Pages/HomeHealthCare.aspx.

17. Albejaidi F, Nair KS. Building the health workforce: Saudi Arabia's challenges in achieving Vision 2030. Int J Health Plann Manage. 2019;34(4):e1405–16. https://doi.org/10.1002/hpm.2861.
18. Alzahrani S. Healthy schools in Saudi Arabia: two decades in review. Int J Pharm Res Allied Sci. 2023;12(1):110–15. https://doi.org/10.51847/lj2fbaa0vm.
19. Centers for Disease Control and Prevention (CDC). School health guidelines to promote healthy eating and physical activity [Internet]. 2011 [cited 2026 Feb 17]. Available from: https://www.cdc.gov/mmwr/pdf/rr/rr6005.pdf.
20. Hilli Y, Pedersen G. School nurses' engagement and care ethics in promoting adolescent health. Nurs Ethics. 2021;28(6):967–79. https://doi.org/10.1177/0969733020985145.
21. General Authority for Statistics (Saudi Arabia). Annual report 2024 [Internet]. 2024 [cited 2026 Feb 17]. Available from: https://www.stats.gov.sa/en/annual-report.
22. Al-Shewear N, Bawazir A. Assessment of school health in Saudi Arabia: the path to improved future students health (implications of the Saudi school health program). J Public Health Dis Prev. 2022;5(1):102.
23. Ministry of Health (Saudi Arabia). Healthy schools [Internet]. 2024 [cited 2026 Feb 17]. Available from: https://www.moh.gov.sa/en/Ministry/Projects/Healthy-Schools/Pages/default.aspx.
24. Aljuaid S, Hazazi H, Bu Mozah A, Haqawi A, Safhi N, Mutanabbik F, et al. The role of nursing in achieving the sustainable development goals of the Kingdom of Saudi Arabia's Vision 2030: systematic literature review. Rev Contemp Philos. 2024;23(2):714–27.
25. Al Asmri M, Almalki MJ, Fitzgerald G, Clark M. The public health care system and primary care services in Saudi Arabia: a system in transition. East Mediterr Health J. 2020;26(4):468–76. https://doi.org/10.26719/emhj.19.049.
26. Al Khashan H, Abogazalah F, Alomary S, Nahhas M, Alwadey A, Al-Khudhair B, et al. Primary health care reform in Saudi Arabia: progress, challenges and prospects. East Mediterr Health J. 2021;27(10):1016–26. https://doi.org/10.26719/emhj.21.042.
27. Alenzi EO, Alqahtani WI, Altwegri MA, Alhelal SM, Alyami WA, Almohana DM, et al. Perceived effectiveness and utilization of health promotion initiatives in Saudi Arabia: insights and recommendations. Healthcare (Basel). 2024;12(23):2352. https://doi.org/10.3390/healthcare12232352.
28. Albejaidi F, Nair K. Nationalisation of health workforce in Saudi Arabia's public and private sectors: a review of issues and challenges. J Health Manag. 2021;23(3):482–97. https://doi.org/10.1177/09720634211035204.
29. Vision 2030 (Saudi Arabia). Health sector transformation program [Internet]. 2025 [cited 2026 Feb 17]. Available from: https://www.vision2030.gov.sa/en/explore/programs/health-sector-transformation-program
30. Almalki A, Al-Hanawi M. Public private partnerships and collaboration in the health sector in the Kingdom of Saudi Arabia: a qualitative study. Glob J Health Sci. 2018;10(6):10–9. https://doi.org/10.5539/gjhs.v10n6p10.
31. Alruwaili M, Ali R, Shahbal S, Alotaibi S, Althiyabi N, Aldosari M, et al. Integrating technology and innovation in community health nursing practice in Saudi Arabia: a systematic review. J Namib Stud Hist Polit Cult. 2023;35:2829–52.
32. Stilwell B. Global health and nursing: a new narrative for the 21st century. 1st ed. Elsevier; 2025.

7 Family as a Client

Learning Objectives

By the end of this chapter, students will be able to:

1. Explain the concept of the family as a client in community health nursing, emphasizing the family as a dynamic, interactive system that influences and is influenced by the health of its members.
2. Analyze diverse family structures, roles, relationships, and communication patterns, and their impact on family health behaviors, decision-making, and overall well-being across different life stages.
3. Apply principles of family assessment using standardized tools such as the genogram, ecomap, Calgary Family Assessment Model (CFAM), Family APGAR, and the McMaster Model of Family Functioning to identify strengths, risks, and health needs.
4. Develop comprehensive and culturally appropriate family-centered care plans that integrate identified health priorities, short- and long-term goals, and evidence-based interventions aligned with Saudi and global health contexts.
5. Implement effective nursing interventions that address health promotion, disease prevention, and rehabilitation within the family unit through education, counseling, coordination, and advocacy.
6. Evaluate family health interventions using measurable indicators related to health outcomes, behavioral changes, family functioning, access to services, and satisfaction, and utilize feedback for continuous improvement.
7. Identify and manage cases of family violence through early detection, risk assessment, crisis intervention, and collaboration with multidisciplinary teams and community protection resources, in accordance with Saudi legal and policy frameworks.

R. I. Ashgar, *Community Health Nursing: Principles, Practices, and Perspectives*,
https://doi.org/10.1007/978-3-032-30791-0_7

8. Discuss the role of support systems—both formal and informal—in promoting family health, and evaluate the community health nurse's function in mobilizing, coordinating, and strengthening these systems.
9. Critically examine the intersection of policy and advocacy in community health nursing practice, and formulate strategies for influencing health policy and promoting equity, safety, and family empowerment.
10. Integrate ethical, cultural, and religious considerations into all aspects of family-centered care to ensure that interventions are respectful, contextually appropriate, and effective within Saudi and global community settings.

Family Health Dynamics

In community health nursing, the family is more than just a unit of individuals—it is a dynamic and interconnected system that influences and is influenced by the health of each member [1]. Recognizing the family as a client shifts the focus from the individual to the collective, enabling community health nurses (CHNs) to promote health and well-being within the context of familial relationships, traditions, and shared environments. In Saudi Arabia, where family ties are deeply rooted in cultural, religious, and social values, this approach holds particular significance. The family unit serves as a primary environment where health behaviors are learned and practiced, making it a critical focus for health interventions [1].

In examining family health dynamics, it is essential to consider the family structure, roles, and relationships, as these elements significantly impact health behaviors and outcomes [2]. Families come in diverse forms, including nuclear, extended, single-parent, and blended families, each with unique health needs and challenges. The roles and responsibilities within a family, such as caregiving and financial support, can affect the physical and mental well-being of its members [3].

Communication patterns within families also play a crucial role in health dynamics. Open and effective communication can facilitate better health management, enabling family members to share health concerns and make informed decisions together. Conversely, poor communication can lead to misunderstandings and inadequate health management, exacerbating health issues [1, 2].

Furthermore, the socioeconomic status of a family influences its access to healthcare resources and services. Families with higher socioeconomic status often have better access to healthcare, nutritious food, and a healthy living environment, which contribute to positive health outcomes. In contrast, families with limited resources may face barriers to accessing healthcare, leading to disparities in health outcomes.

Cultural beliefs and practices within a family also shape health behaviors and attitudes towards healthcare. Cultural norms can influence dietary habits, health-seeking behavior, and adherence to medical advice [4]. CHNs must be culturally competent to effectively engage with families from diverse backgrounds, respecting their beliefs while promoting healthy practices.

The life cycle stage of the family further affects health dynamics. For instance, families with young children may focus on immunizations and nutrition, while those with elderly members may prioritize chronic disease management and mobility issues. Understanding the specific needs at each life cycle stage allows for tailored health interventions that address the unique challenges faced by families [5].

Stress and coping mechanisms within families are additional factors influencing health dynamics. Families encountering high levels of stress, whether from financial difficulties, health crises, or interpersonal conflicts, may experience negative health outcomes. Effective coping strategies, such as social support and problem-solving skills, can mitigate the impact of stress on family health [5, 6].

CHNs play a vital role in assessing and enhancing family health dynamics. Through home visits, health education, and advocacy, nurses can identify health risks, promote healthy behaviors, and connect families with community resources. By adopting a holistic approach that considers the family as a unit, CHNs can foster environments that support optimal health for all family members [3].

In conclusion, understanding family health dynamics is essential for developing effective community health interventions. By recognizing the diverse factors that influence family health, healthcare professionals can design strategies that promote wellness and prevent disease, ultimately improving the health outcomes of families within the community.

Family Assessment Tools

Family assessment tools are integral in understanding the dynamics, strengths, and needs of families within the context of community health nursing. These tools provide a structured framework for nurses to collect comprehensive data about family structure, function, and development, which are essential in planning and delivering effective care [2, 5].

One of the key tools used in family assessment is the genogram (Fig. 7.1). A genogram is a graphical representation that maps out the family structure and provides detailed information about the relationships and health patterns within the family. It includes data on at least three generations, offering insights into hereditary conditions and psychosocial issues. This tool helps nurses identify patterns of illnesses, such as genetic disorders, and understand family dynamics that might affect health behaviors and outcomes [2].

Another important tool is the ecomap (Fig. 7.2), which complements the genogram by illustrating the family's interactions with external systems. An ecomap provides a visual representation of the family's connections to social networks, community resources, and support systems. This helps nurses assess the level of support available to the family and identify potential stressors or resources that can be leveraged to improve health outcomes [2].

The Calgary Family Assessment Model (CFAM) is a comprehensive framework that guides the assessment of families (Fig. 7.3). It encompasses three major categories: structural, developmental, and functional assessments. The structural assessment

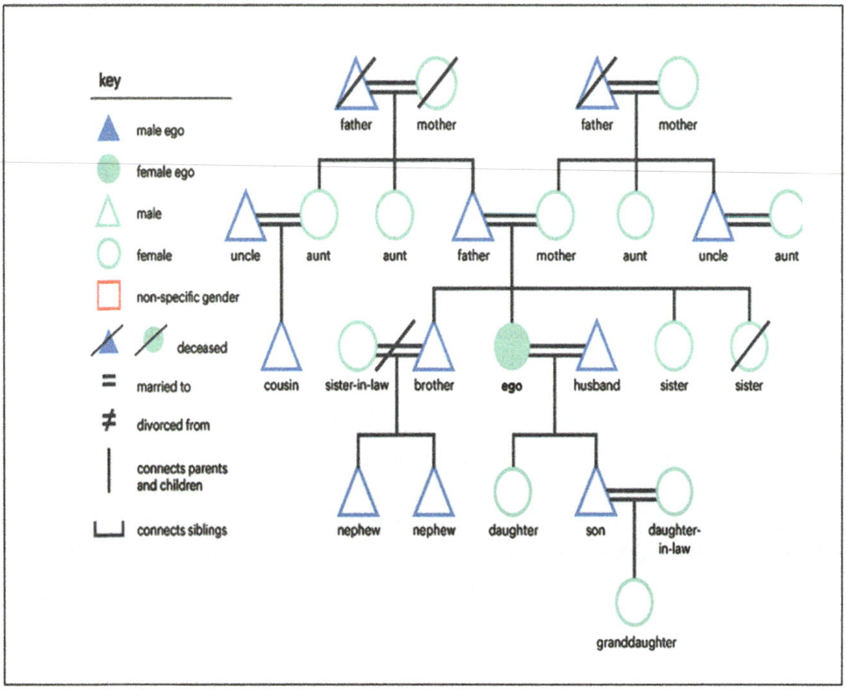

Fig. 7.1 Family genogram

focuses on who is in the family, the relationships among them, and other individuals or institutions that influence the family. The developmental assessment considers the family's life cycle and the transitions they are experiencing. Functional assessment explores how family members interact and communicate with each other, including problem-solving abilities, roles, and emotional support [7].

Family APGAR is a simple but effective tool used to assess family function. It consists of five parameters: Adaptability, Partnership, Growth, Affection, and Resolve. Each parameter is scored to provide an overall picture of family satisfaction and functioning. This tool is particularly useful for quickly identifying families that may require more in-depth assessment or intervention [8].

The McMaster Model of Family Functioning is another framework used to evaluate the family's health and functioning (see Fig. 7.4). This model assesses six dimensions of family life: problem solving, communication, roles, affective responsiveness, affective involvement, and behavior control. By examining these areas, nurses can identify strengths and areas for improvement, facilitating targeted interventions to enhance family functioning [9].

Incorporating these tools into community health nursing practice allows for a holistic approach to care, recognizing the family as a central unit of health. These assessments provide critical insights that inform the development of personalized

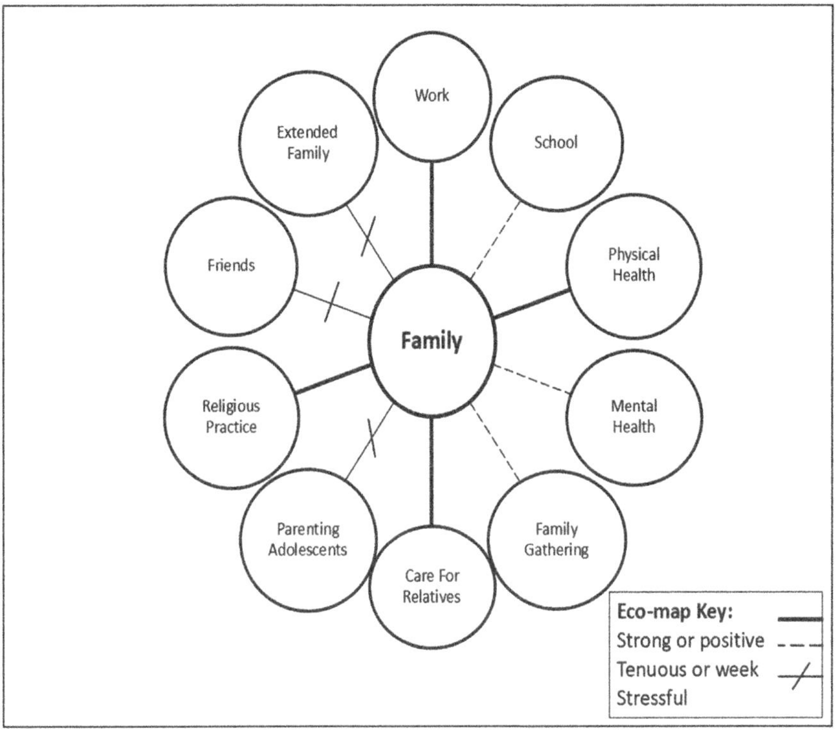

Fig. 7.2 Family ecomap

Table 7.1 Family APGAR domains

Components	
Adaptation	Adaptation refers to the strategic use of family resources to address and manage challenges arising from life changes that threaten the stability or equilibrium of the family system.
Partnership	Partnership within the family refers to the collaborative involvement of members in decision-making processes and the shared responsibility for providing care and support.
Growth	Growth refers to the physical and emotional development, as well as the pursuit of self-fulfillment, attained by family members through reciprocal support and guidance.
Affection	Affection is the caring or loving relationship that exists among family members.
Resolve	Resolve is the commitment to allocating family resources toward the physical and emotional care and support of other family members.

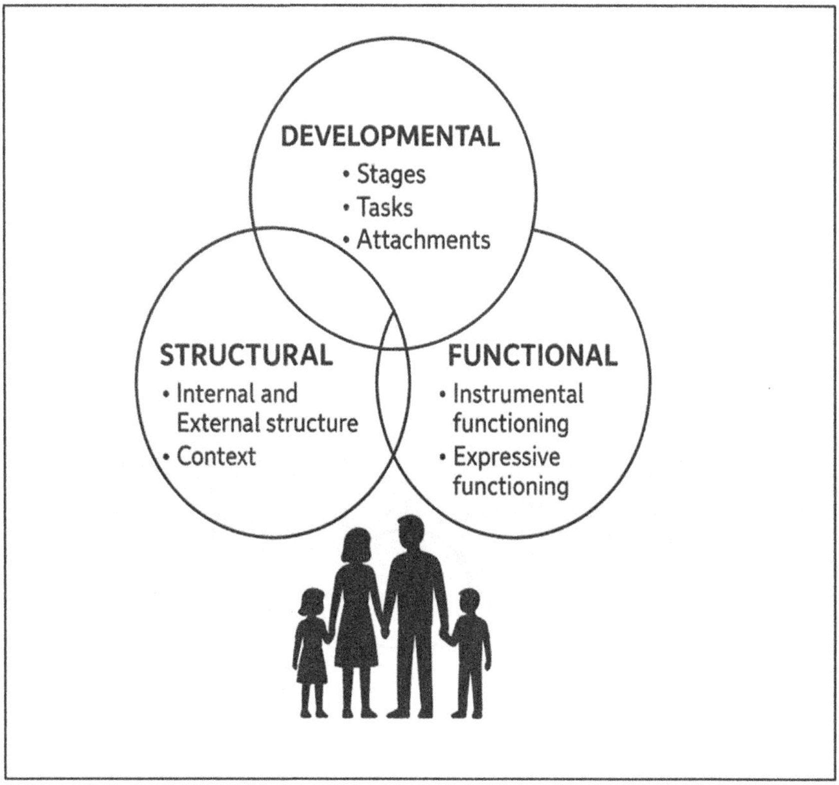

Fig. 7.3 Calgary Family Assessment Model (CFAM)

care plans, promote family engagement, and ultimately improve health outcomes. Furthermore, they emphasize the importance of cultural respect, as understanding and respecting cultural differences is essential in accurately assessing and addressing family needs. By using these tools, nurses can better support families in navigating health challenges and achieving optimal health and well-being [2].

Planning and Implementation of Care

Once the family has been assessed as a unit, the next critical steps in community health nursing are planning and implementing care that addresses their specific health needs. These stages are grounded in a partnership approach, recognizing the family's autonomy, values, culture, and capacity for change [1].

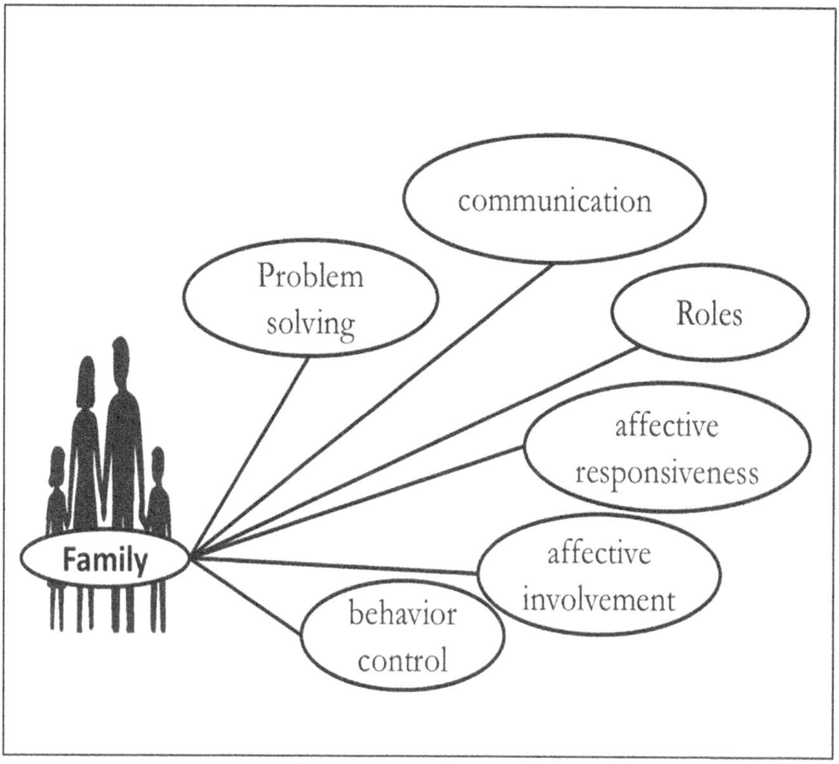

Fig. 7.4 McMaster Model of Family Functioning

A. Planning of Care

Effective planning ensures that nursing interventions are goal-oriented, family-centered, and culturally appropriate.

1. **Setting Priorities**
   - Nurses work collaboratively with families to identify and prioritize health needs.
   - Priority is given to issues that:
     - Threaten life or function (e.g., chronic illness, child malnutrition).
     - Are preventable or manageable with education or support.
     - Have been identified as important by the family themselves.
2. **Establishing Goals and Objectives**
   - **Short-term goals** may focus on managing current symptoms or improving health behaviors (e.g., "Mother will monitor her blood pressure daily for two weeks").

- **Long-term goals** address sustained family wellness (e.g., "The family will adopt a balanced dietary plan to manage diabetes and prevent obesity in children").

3. **Selecting Interventions**
   - Interventions are tailored to the family's structure, resources, literacy level, and readiness for change.
   - Examples include:
     - Health education sessions (e.g., on nutrition, breastfeeding, medication adherence).
     - Behavioral interventions (e.g., smoking cessation, increasing physical activity).
     - Resource mobilization (e.g., referrals to social workers or financial aid programs).

4. **Cultural and Religious Considerations**
   - Plans must be compatible with religious values, such as preferences for same-gender healthcare providers, dietary restrictions (e.g., halal food), and observance of religious practices such as prayer and fasting.
   - Involvement of extended family members may be necessary in decision-making.

B. Implementation of Care

This phase involves putting the care plan into action using evidence-based interventions while remaining flexible to the family's circumstances and feedback.

1. **Health Education and Promotion**
   - Delivered during home visits, community clinics, or health campaigns.
   - Topics may include:
     - Disease prevention (e.g., vaccinations, hygiene, genetic counseling).
     - Chronic disease management (e.g., diabetes, hypertension).
     - Mental health awareness and destigmatization.

2. **Supportive Counseling and Advocacy**
   - Nurses provide emotional and psychological support to families dealing with:
     - Grief and loss.
     - Disabilities or chronic illness.
     - Family conflict or caregiving stress.
   - Nurses may also act as advocates, linking families to housing, food support, or disability services.

3. **Coordination of Services**
   - CHNs often act as care coordinators, especially for families with complex health needs.

- They liaise with:
  - Physicians and specialists.
  - School health services.
  - Social workers and religious leaders.

4. **Monitoring and Follow-Up**
   - Continued engagement is critical to evaluate progress and adapt interventions.
   - Regular home visits or follow-up calls are scheduled to:
     - Reassess health status.
     - Reinforce education.
     - Ensure medication and treatment compliance.

Example in a Saudi Context

A nurse visits a rural Saudi family where the father has uncontrolled diabetes, and the teenage daughter shows early signs of depression. After assessing the family's needs and dynamics, the nurse develops a care plan that includes dietary education for the mother (primary caregiver), coordination with a PHC to encourage the father's participation in group health sessions, and a telehealth referral to a psychologist for the daughter. Follow-up visits are scheduled every 2 weeks to support adherence and adjust interventions as needed.

Challenges in Implementation

- **Limited resources** in rural areas or underserved neighborhoods.
- **Language barriers** with non-Arabic-speaking family members or caregivers.
- **Health literacy gaps** affecting understanding of disease and treatment.
- **Stigma** associated with certain conditions such as mental health or disability.

CHNs must use flexible, culturally sensitive approaches to overcome these challenges and ensure that care remains effective and respectful.

Evaluation of Family Health Interventions

Evaluation is the final but ongoing phase of the nursing process. It involves systematically determining whether the planned family health interventions have been effective in achieving desired outcomes. In community health nursing—particularly when families are the focus—evaluation goes beyond individual health status to encompass family dynamics, functioning, satisfaction, and health behavior change.

Evaluation of family health interventions may focus on various dimensions:

a. Health Outcomes

- Improvements in physical or mental health (e.g., blood pressure control, diabetes management, vaccination rates).
- Reduction in hospital admissions or emergency room visits.
- Successful completion of treatment regimens.

b. Behavioral Changes

- Adoption of healthy behaviors (e.g., diet, exercise, medication adherence).
- Reduction in harmful behaviors (e.g., smoking, sedentary lifestyle).
- Improved parenting practices or elder care routines.

c. Family Function and Support

- Enhanced communication within the family.
- Greater participation in care planning and health promotion.
- Strengthened caregiving roles and support systems.

d. Access and Utilization of Services

- Increased use of preventive and primary care services.
- Engagement with community health resources (e.g., home visits, telehealth, school health services).

e. Client and Family Satisfaction

- Feedback on the clarity, usefulness, and cultural sensitivity of care.
- Satisfaction with nurse–family interactions and follow-up.
- Perceived improvements in quality of life.

Family Violence

The prevalence of family violence presents significant challenges to community health nursing, requiring multifaceted interventions to address its complex nature. Health professionals play a critical role in the identification, prevention, and management of family violence, necessitating a comprehensive and interdisciplinary approach. Effective interventions encompass a range of strategies, including early identification, risk assessment, crisis intervention, and long-term support [6, 10].

Early identification of family violence is crucial, as it allows for timely intervention and prevention of further harm. Health professionals must be adept at recognizing the subtle signs of abuse, which may include physical injuries, psychological distress, or social withdrawal. Training in effective communication and observational skills is essential for nurses to identify potential cases of family violence. Furthermore, creating a safe and confidential environment encourages individuals to disclose their experiences without fear of judgment or retaliation.

Risk assessment is another vital component of interventions for family violence. This involves evaluating the severity and frequency of violence, the potential for escalation, and the presence of protective factors. Standardized tools and protocols can aid health professionals in systematically assessing risk and determining the appropriate level of intervention. By understanding the dynamics of abuse and the specific needs of those affected, nurses can tailor their interventions to ensure the safety and well-being of victims.

Crisis intervention is often necessary when dealing with acute cases of family violence. This involves providing immediate support and stabilization to individuals in distress. Health professionals must be skilled in de-escalation techniques and crisis management to effectively handle volatile situations. Collaboration with law enforcement and social services is also crucial in ensuring the safety of victims and facilitating access to emergency resources.

Long-term support is critical for survivors of family violence to rebuild their lives and achieve lasting recovery. This includes providing access to counseling services, support groups, and educational programs that empower individuals to regain control and independence. Health professionals play a pivotal role in coordinating care and connecting survivors with community resources that address their physical, emotional, and social needs.

Moreover, community health nursing interventions should incorporate a public health perspective, focusing on prevention and education. This involves raising awareness about the signs of family violence and promoting healthy relationship dynamics through community outreach programs. Engaging community leaders and stakeholders in these efforts enhances the effectiveness and sustainability of prevention initiatives.

Interdisciplinary collaboration is essential in addressing the multifaceted nature of family violence. Health professionals, social workers, legal advocates, and educators must work together to create a network of support for individuals and families affected by violence. By fostering partnerships across sectors, CHNs can contribute to the development of comprehensive strategies that address the root causes of family violence and promote a culture of safety and respect.

In conclusion, interventions for family violence within community health nursing require a holistic and collaborative approach. By prioritizing early identification, risk assessment, crisis intervention, and long-term support, health professionals can effectively address the complex needs of individuals affected by family violence and contribute to the overall health and well-being of the community.

Legal and Policy Framework in Saudi Arabia

Saudi Arabia has implemented several measures to combat family violence:

- **Protection from Abuse Law (2013):** Criminalizes abuse and outlines penalties [11].
- **Family Protection Centers:** Safe spaces for victims across the Kingdom.
- **Human Rights Commission:** Ensures victims' rights and monitors compliance.
- **Vision 2030 Social Reforms:** Promote gender equality, women's participation, and child protection.

Healthcare providers are legally obligated to report suspected abuse to authorities such as the MOH or the Ministry of Human Resources and Social Development.

Support Systems

Support systems play a crucial role in the domain of community health nursing, providing essential resources and networks that enhance healthcare delivery and patient outcomes. These systems encompass a broad spectrum of services and structures designed to assist individuals, families, and communities in maintaining and improving health.

At the core of support systems in community health nursing is the integration of formal and informal networks. Formal support systems include healthcare institutions, governmental health agencies, and non-governmental organizations that offer structured health services and programs. These entities provide critical healthcare interventions, ranging from preventive services to acute care, ensuring that communities have access to essential health resources. Informal support systems, on the other hand, consist of family, friends, and community groups that offer emotional, social, and practical support. The synergy between formal and informal systems is vital for creating a comprehensive support network that addresses diverse health needs.

CHNs play a pivotal role in facilitating and coordinating these support systems. They act as liaisons between patients and healthcare services, ensuring that individuals receive appropriate and timely care. By assessing the unique needs of the community, nurses can identify gaps in existing support structures and advocate for necessary resources. This advocacy often involves collaborating with local organizations to develop programs that address specific health challenges, such as chronic disease management, maternal and child health, and elder care.

Furthermore, support systems in community health nursing are increasingly incorporating technology to enhance service delivery. Telehealth and mobile health applications provide innovative solutions for reaching underserved populations, offering remote consultations, health education, and monitoring services. These technological advancements not only improve access to care but also empower individuals to take an active role in managing their health.

Education and training are also integral components of effective support systems. CHNs engage in continuous professional development to stay abreast of current healthcare practices and policies. They also play a key role in educating the community about health promotion and disease prevention strategies. By fostering a culture of health literacy, nurses empower individuals to make informed health decisions, thereby strengthening the overall support system.

Moreover, policy and advocacy efforts are essential for sustaining and expanding support systems in community health nursing. Nurses often participate in policy-making processes to influence healthcare legislation and funding allocations. By advocating for policies that prioritize community health needs, they help to secure the necessary resources and infrastructure to support comprehensive healthcare delivery.

In summary, support systems are a fundamental aspect of community health nursing, providing the framework for effective healthcare delivery and improved health outcomes. Through the integration of formal and informal networks, the incorporation of technology, and ongoing education and advocacy efforts, these systems ensure that communities are equipped to meet their health needs. CHNs, as key facilitators of these systems, play a crucial role in bridging the gap between healthcare services and the populations they serve, ultimately contributing to the health and well-being of the community.

Policy and Advocacy

In the realm of community health nursing, the integration of policy and advocacy plays a pivotal role in shaping health outcomes and advancing public health objectives. This subchapter delves into the strategic incorporation of policy frameworks and advocacy efforts that CHNs employ to influence health systems and promote equitable health practices.

Community health nursing professionals are uniquely positioned to act as intermediaries between the healthcare system and the community. Their comprehensive understanding of community dynamics allows them to effectively identify health disparities and advocate for policies that address these inequities. By engaging in policy development, nurses contribute to the creation of health policies that are responsive to the needs of diverse populations. This involvement not only enhances the quality of care provided but also ensures that healthcare delivery systems are more inclusive and equitable [10].

The advocacy role of CHNs involves a multifaceted approach, encompassing direct patient advocacy, community engagement, and policy advocacy at local, state, and national levels. Direct patient advocacy involves supporting individual patients in navigating the healthcare system and ensuring they receive appropriate care and resources. This aspect of advocacy is crucial in empowering patients and fostering a sense of agency in their health management [3, 4].

At the community level, health nurses engage in advocacy by collaborating with community leaders and organizations to address public health issues. This collaboration often involves educating the community about health risks and preventive measures, thereby enhancing public health literacy. Moreover, CHNs facilitate community involvement in health decision-making processes, ensuring that community voices are heard in policy formulation.

On a broader scale, policy advocacy involves influencing legislation and public policy to create a supportive environment for health promotion. CHNs participate in policy advocacy by joining professional organizations, attending policy forums, and engaging with policymakers. Their firsthand experience and insights into community health challenges make them invaluable contributors to policy discussions. By articulating the health needs and concerns of the communities they serve, nurses can influence policy decisions that lead to improved health outcomes.

Furthermore, CHNs leverage data and research to support their advocacy efforts. By utilizing evidence-based practices, they provide compelling arguments for policy changes that are grounded in scientific research. This approach not only strengthens their advocacy efforts but also enhances the credibility of their recommendations in the eyes of policymakers.

In summary, the integration of policy and advocacy within community health nursing is essential for advancing public health goals and promoting health equity. Through their advocacy efforts, CHNs play a critical role in shaping health policies that reflect the needs and priorities of the communities they serve. Their ability to influence policy and advocate for systemic change underscores the importance of their role in the healthcare ecosystem. As the landscape of public health continues to evolve, the advocacy and policy contributions of CHNs will remain indispensable in driving progress and ensuring health equity for all.

References

1. Robinson M, Coehlo D, Smith P. Family health care nursing: theory, practice, and research. 7th ed. F.A. Davis Company; 2022.
2. Shajan Z, Snell D. Wright & Leahey's nurses and families: a guide to family assessment and intervention. F.A. Davis; 2019.
3. Nies MA, McEwen M. Community/public health nursing: promoting the health of populations. 8th ed. Elsevier; 2023.
4. Stanhope M, Lancaster J. Public health nursing: population-centered health care in the community. 11th ed. Elsevier; 2024.
5. McCubbin HI, Thompson AI, McCubbin MA. Family assessment: resiliency, coping and adaptation—inventories for research and practice. University of Wisconsin; 1996.
6. Herdiana I, Suryanto S, Handoyo S. Family resilience: a conceptual review. Adv Soc Sci Educ Humanit Res. 2018;133:42–8. https://doi.org/10.2991/acpch-17.2018.9.
7. Mileski M, McClay R, Heinemann K, Dray G. Efficacy of the use of the Calgary Family Intervention Model in bedside nursing education: a systematic review. J Multidiscip Healthc. 2022;15:1323–47. https://doi.org/10.2147/JMDH.S370053.
8. Smilkstein G. The family APGAR: a proposal for a family function test and its use by physicians. J Fam Pract. 1978;6(6):1231–39.
9. Miller IW, Ryan CE, Keitner GI, Bishop DS, Epstein NB. The McMaster approach to families: theory, assessment, treatment, and research. J Fam Ther. 2000;22:168–89.
10. Barnes MD, Hanson CL, Novilla LB, Magnusson BM, Crandall AC, Bradford G. Family-centered health promotion: perspectives for engaging families and achieving better health outcomes. Inquiry. 2020;57:46958020923537. https://doi.org/10.1177/0046958020923537.
11. Ministry of Human Resources and Social Development (Saudi Arabia). Executive regulation of the law of protection from abuse [Internet]. 2017 [cited 2026 Feb 17]. Available from: https://www.hrsd.gov.sa/en/knowledge-centre/decisions-and-regulations/regulation-and-procedures/70781

Community Health Education

8

Learning Objectives

By the end of this chapter, students will be able to:

1. Explain the fundamental principles and goals of health education within the context of community health nursing, emphasizing its role in disease prevention, health promotion, and behavior change.
2. Analyze the determinants of health behaviors—including cultural, socioeconomic, and demographic factors—and their implications for planning and delivering effective health education interventions.
3. Conduct a comprehensive needs assessment to identify the health priorities, resources, and challenges of a community, forming the evidence base for targeted health education programs.
4. Design health education programs using systematic approaches that include goal setting, formulation of SMART objectives, selection of evidence-based strategies, and integration of appropriate learning theories.
5. Apply principles of effective communication and adult learning to implement culturally and linguistically appropriate health education interventions across diverse populations and settings.
6. Incorporate technology—including digital media, telehealth, and mobile health applications—into health education initiatives to enhance accessibility, engagement, and sustainability of learning outcomes.
7. Demonstrate skills in community engagement and partnership-building by involving stakeholders, local organizations, and community leaders in the design, implementation, and evaluation of health programs.
8. Evaluate the effectiveness of health education programs using both formative and summative evaluation methods, assessing changes in knowledge, attitudes, behaviors, and health outcomes at the individual and community levels.

R. I. Ashgar, *Community Health Nursing: Principles, Practices, and Perspectives*,
https://doi.org/10.1007/978-3-032-30791-0_8

9. Critically appraise available health education resources (national, international, and digital) for credibility, cultural appropriateness, and applicability in promoting health literacy and equity.
10. Advocate for health-promoting policies and public health initiatives that address social determinants of health, reduce disparities, and sustain community empowerment through education.

Principles of Health Education

Health education is a vital component of community health nursing, serving as the cornerstone for promoting health and preventing disease. It encompasses a strategic approach to empowering individuals and communities with the knowledge, skills, and motivation necessary to make informed health decisions [1]. The principles of health education are grounded in a systematic process that includes assessing needs, planning effective interventions, implementing strategies, and evaluating outcomes [1].

The primary goal of health education is to foster an environment where individuals and communities can achieve optimal health. This begins with a comprehensive assessment of the community's health needs. Understanding the demographic, cultural, and socioeconomic factors that influence health behaviors is essential. This assessment phase lays the foundation for developing targeted educational interventions that are culturally sensitive and relevant [2].

Planning is the next critical step in health education. It involves setting clear, achievable objectives that align with the overall health goals of the community. Health educators must design programs that are evidence-based and tailored to the specific needs of the population. This requires a thorough understanding of the health issues at hand and the factors that contribute to them. Engaging community members in the planning process ensures that the programs are relevant and sustainable [3, 4].

Implementation of health education strategies requires the use of effective communication techniques. Health educators must employ a variety of methods to disseminate information, including workshops, seminars, digital media, and one-on-one counseling. The choice of method depends on the target audience and the complexity of the health message. Interactive and participatory approaches are often more effective in facilitating behavior change, as they encourage active involvement and personal investment in the learning process [5, 6].

Evaluation is a fundamental principle of health education, providing a mechanism for assessing the effectiveness of educational interventions. This involves measuring changes in knowledge, attitudes, and behaviors among the target population. Evaluation helps to identify successful strategies and areas for improvement, ensuring that health education programs remain dynamic and responsive to the changing needs of the community [7].

Health education is not a one-size-fits-all approach; it requires adaptation to the unique characteristics of each community. Cultural respect is crucial in this regard, as it enables health educators to respect and incorporate diverse cultural beliefs and practices into their programs. Building trust and rapport with community members is essential for overcoming barriers to education and fostering a supportive environment for learning [1].

In addition to individual and community-level interventions, health education also plays a role in influencing public policy. By advocating for health-promoting policies and practices, health educators can help create environments that support healthy choices and behaviors. This advocacy is an extension of the educational process, aiming to address the broader determinants of health and reduce health disparities. Overall, the principles of health education emphasize the importance of a comprehensive, collaborative, and culturally sensitive approach to health promotion. By empowering individuals and communities with the knowledge and skills needed to make informed health decisions, health education contributes to the overall well-being and resilience of communities.

Designing Educational Programs

In the field of community health nursing, the development of educational programs is fundamental to enhancing public health. This process involves a systematic approach that is rooted in theory and practice, ensuring that the educational interventions are effective and sustainable [8, 9]. The initial phase of designing educational programs involves conducting a thorough needs assessment. This assessment identifies the specific health needs of the community, considering factors such as demographic characteristics, prevalent health issues, and available resources. By understanding these elements, health professionals can tailor their educational programs to address the most pressing needs effectively.

Subsequent to the needs assessment, setting clear and measurable objectives becomes paramount. These objectives should align with the overall goals of the community health initiative and should be specific, measurable, achievable, relevant, and time-bound (SMART). Clearly defined objectives provide a roadmap for the educational program and facilitate the evaluation of its effectiveness [6].

The selection of educational strategies is a critical step in the program design. Strategies should be evidence-based and culturally appropriate, taking into account the literacy levels and learning preferences of the target audience. Interactive methods such as workshops, group discussions, and role-playing are often more effective than traditional didactic approaches, as they engage participants actively and foster a deeper understanding of the material [8].

Incorporating technology into educational programs can also enhance learning outcomes. Digital tools such as mobile applications, online courses, and social media platforms can be leveraged to disseminate information widely and facilitate continuous learning. These tools are particularly useful in reaching diverse populations and overcoming geographical barriers. Furthermore, collaboration with community stakeholders is essential in the program design process. Engaging local leaders, healthcare providers, and community organizations ensures that the program is relevant and supported by the community. This collaboration fosters a sense of ownership among participants, which can enhance the program's sustainability [2, 4].

Evaluation is an integral part of designing educational programs. It involves assessing both the process and the outcomes of the program to determine its effectiveness and identify areas for improvement. Formative evaluation, conducted during the program, provides immediate feedback and allows for adjustments to be made in real-time. Summative evaluation, conducted after the program's completion, measures the overall impact and informs future program planning [10].

In summary, designing educational programs in community health nursing requires a comprehensive and collaborative approach. By conducting a needs assessment, setting clear objectives, selecting appropriate strategies, leveraging technology, and engaging stakeholders, health professionals can develop effective educational interventions that improve community health outcomes. Continuous evaluation ensures that these programs remain relevant and impactful, ultimately contributing to the enhancement of public health.

Implementation Strategies

The effective implementation of community health nursing strategies necessitates a multifaceted approach, integrating evidence-based practices with culturally sensitive interventions that address the unique needs of diverse populations [8]. Central to these strategies is the establishment of a collaborative framework that engages stakeholders at various levels—ranging from individual clients to community leaders and policymakers.

A critical component of implementation is the assessment and utilization of community resources. This involves conducting comprehensive community health assessments to identify existing resources, gaps, and potential barriers to care. By leveraging local assets and fostering partnerships with community organizations, healthcare providers can enhance service delivery and ensure that interventions are sustainable and responsive to community needs.

Integration of technology plays a pivotal role in modern implementation strategies. The use of electronic health records (EHRs), telehealth services, and mobile health applications facilitates improved communication, data collection, and monitoring of health outcomes. These technological tools enable healthcare providers to deliver personalized care, track patient progress in real-time, and engage clients in their health management processes.

Cultural respect is another cornerstone of successful implementation. Healthcare providers must be equipped with the skills and knowledge to deliver culturally appropriate care, recognizing and respecting the diverse values, beliefs, and practices of the populations they serve. This includes the incorporation of traditional health practices where appropriate, and the adaptation of health education materials and interventions to align with cultural norms and languages.

Community engagement is vital for the successful adoption and sustainability of health interventions. Strategies should emphasize the active participation of community members in the planning, implementation, and evaluation of health programs. This participatory approach ensures that interventions are tailored to the specific needs and preferences of the community, thereby enhancing acceptability and effectiveness.

Moreover, continuous evaluation and quality improvement processes are essential to refine and optimize implementation strategies. Utilizing both qualitative and quantitative data, healthcare providers can assess the impact of interventions, identify areas for improvement, and make necessary adjustments to enhance outcomes. This iterative process fosters a culture of learning and adaptability, which is crucial in the dynamic field of community health nursing.

The development of interdisciplinary teams is also a key strategy in implementation. By bringing together professionals from various disciplines—such as nursing, social work, nutrition, and public health—teams can provide holistic care that addresses the physical, emotional, and social determinants of health. This collaborative approach not only enhances the quality of care but also promotes the efficient use of resources.

Finally, advocacy and policy development are integral to the implementation of community health nursing strategies. Nurses and other healthcare professionals must engage in advocacy efforts to influence health policy, secure funding, and promote systemic changes that support health equity and access to care. Through active participation in policy-making processes, healthcare providers can help shape an environment that facilitates the successful implementation of community health initiatives.

Evaluation of Outcomes

In the realm of community health nursing, the evaluation of outcomes is a critical component that ensures the effectiveness of healthcare interventions and strategies. The process of evaluating outcomes involves a systematic assessment of the results of health programs and interventions implemented within a community. This evaluation is essential for determining the impact of nursing care on the health status of the population served [11, 12]. By analyzing these outcomes, healthcare providers can identify the strengths and weaknesses of their interventions, allowing for continuous improvement and adaptation to meet the evolving needs of the community.

Outcome evaluation in community health nursing encompasses several key dimensions, including the measurement of health status improvements, behavioral changes, and the accessibility and quality of healthcare services. Health status improvements are often measured through changes in morbidity and mortality rates, prevalence of diseases, and overall community health indicators. These metrics provide quantitative data that reflect the effectiveness of health interventions in reducing disease burden and enhancing the well-being of individuals and communities.

Behavioral changes are another critical aspect of outcome evaluation. These changes can be observed in the adoption of healthier lifestyles, increased health literacy, and improved self-care practices among community members. Evaluating behavioral outcomes helps in understanding the extent to which health education and promotion activities have influenced individuals' choices and actions regarding their health. Such evaluations are crucial for tailoring future health education programs to better address the specific needs and challenges faced by the community.

The accessibility and quality of healthcare services are also vital components of outcome evaluation. Access to healthcare is measured by assessing the availability, affordability, and acceptability of health services to the community. Quality of care, on the other hand, is evaluated through patient satisfaction surveys, adherence to clinical guidelines, and the effectiveness of care delivery processes. By examining these factors, community health nurses can identify barriers to healthcare access and areas for quality improvement, ultimately enhancing the overall healthcare experience for community members.

Moreover, the evaluation of outcomes in community health nursing is not only limited to health-related metrics but also includes the assessment of economic and social impacts. Economic evaluations consider the cost-effectiveness of health interventions, analyzing the financial resources invested in relation to the health benefits achieved. Social impact assessments focus on the broader effects of health programs on community empowerment, social cohesion, and equity. These evaluations provide a comprehensive understanding of the value and implications of health interventions beyond immediate health outcomes.

To effectively evaluate outcomes, community health nurses employ a variety of methods and tools, including surveys, interviews, focus groups, and health data analysis. These methods facilitate the collection of both qualitative and quantitative data, offering a holistic view of the intervention outcomes. Collaboration with community stakeholders, including patients, families, and local organizations, is also essential in the outcome evaluation process. Engaging stakeholders ensures that the evaluation is culturally sensitive and aligned with the community's values and priorities.

In conclusion, the evaluation of outcomes is an integral part of community health nursing that informs evidence-based practice and policy development. By systematically assessing the impact of health interventions, community health nurses can enhance the effectiveness of their care, contribute to the improvement of population health, and ensure the sustainability of health programs. This ongoing process of evaluation and adaptation is crucial for addressing the dynamic health needs of communities and achieving the overarching goals of public health.

Community Engagement

Community engagement within the realm of community health nursing is a pivotal element that fosters collaboration between healthcare providers and the community. This partnership is essential for identifying health priorities and developing strategies to address them effectively. The engagement process involves active participation from community members, which not only empowers them but also ensures that health interventions are culturally appropriate and sustainable [3].

The foundation of community engagement lies in understanding the unique characteristics and needs of the community. This involves conducting comprehensive community assessments to gather data on health status, resources, and social determinants of health. Such assessments provide valuable insights that guide the development of tailored interventions aimed at improving health outcomes.

A key aspect of community engagement is the establishment of trust and mutual respect between healthcare providers and community members. Building trust requires transparency in communication and decision-making processes, as well as a genuine commitment to addressing the community's concerns. Healthcare providers must be adept at listening to the voices of the community, acknowledging their experiences, and incorporating their feedback into health programs.

Community engagement also emphasizes the importance of collaboration across various sectors, including education, local government, and non-profit organizations. This multi-sectoral approach leverages diverse resources and expertise, creating a comprehensive framework for addressing complex health issues. Collaborative efforts can lead to the development of community coalitions that advocate for health policies and programs, enhancing the overall impact of community health initiatives.

Furthermore, community engagement involves capacity building, which equips community members with the knowledge and skills necessary to take an active role in health promotion. Through educational workshops and training sessions, community members can become health advocates, spreading awareness and encouraging healthy behaviors among their peers.

The evaluation of community engagement efforts is crucial to determine their effectiveness and identify areas for improvement. This involves setting measurable objectives and utilizing both qualitative and quantitative methods to assess outcomes. Feedback from community members is integral to this process, as it provides insights into the perceived impact of health interventions and highlights any challenges encountered.

In community health nursing, the role of the nurse extends beyond traditional healthcare delivery. Nurses act as facilitators of community engagement, bridging the gap between healthcare systems and the community. They are instrumental in initiating dialogues, fostering partnerships, and advocating for resources that address the social determinants of health. Ultimately, community engagement is a dynamic and ongoing process that requires continuous effort and adaptation. It is not a one-size-fits-all approach, but rather a tailored strategy that evolves with the changing needs of the community. By prioritizing community engagement, community health nursing can effectively address health disparities and promote health equity, leading to healthier and more resilient communities.

Health Education Resources

A wide array of health education materials, media, and resources is readily available through both national and international health organizations, governmental agencies, and non-governmental entities. These resources encompass print formats—such as brochures, pamphlets, posters, and booklets—as well as digital and electronic formats, including interactive websites, mobile applications, videos, and e-learning modules. Many of these materials are accessible to the public either free of charge or at a minimal cost, ensuring that essential health information can reach diverse populations regardless of socioeconomic status.

Community health nurses (CHNs) play a critical role in bridging the gap between these resources and the populations they serve. By staying informed about the availability, credibility, and cultural appropriateness of health education tools, nurses can guide individuals, families, and groups in locating and utilizing appropriate educational content. Additionally, CHNs can connect clients to local services such as community health centers, support groups, wellness programs, or equipment loan services (e.g., mobility aids, blood pressure monitors). In doing so, they empower communities with the knowledge and tools necessary for informed decision-making and proactive health management. Nurses' awareness of local, regional, and national resources enhances their ability to deliver person-centered care and promote health equity across diverse settings. Some examples of health education resources are:

- Regional hospitals, clinics, and libraries.
- Governmental sources (e.g., Ministry of Health website, Health Education page [13]).
- Saudi Digital Library [14].
- Universities and colleges.
- Professional organizations (e.g., American Public Health Association, Society for Behavioral Medicine)

Commercial organizations (e.g., pharmaceutical companies and medical supply companies).

References

1. Bastable SB. Nurse as educator: principles of teaching and learning for nursing practice. Jones & Bartlett Learning; 2021.
2. Anderson ET, McFarlane J. Community as partner: theory and practice in nursing. 8th ed. Lippincott Williams & Wilkins; 2018.
3. Michener JL, Williams A, Oto-Kent D, Aguilar-Gaxiola S. Community engagement: a foundation for health equity and resilience. Am J Public Health. 2025;115(Suppl):S104–9. https://doi.org/10.2105/AJPH.2025.308029.
4. World Health Organization (WHO). Community engagement for quality health services [Internet]. 2025 [cited 2026 Feb 17]. Available from: https://www.who.int/teams/integrated-health-services/quality-of-care/community-engagement
5. Ashgar R. Community-based participatory research in cardiovascular disease prevention for middle-aged women: a systematic review. Heart Int. 2025;19(1):12–9. https://doi.org/10.17925/HI.2025.19.1.1.
6. Kim DKD, Kreps GL, Singhal A. Health communication: strategies for developing global health programs. Peter Lang; 2014.
7. Murdaugh CL, Parsons MA, Pender NJ. Health promotion in nursing practice. 8th ed. Pearson; 2018.
8. Alazwari I, Alarsan S, Alkhateeb N, Salameh E. Designing effective health education programs: a review of current research and best practices. Int J Med Res Health Sci. 2023;12(2):42–6.
9. DeMarco RF, Healey-Walsh J. Community & public health nursing: evidence for practice. 3rd ed. Lippincott Williams & Wilkins; 2020.

10. Salazar LF, Crosby RA, DiClemente RJ. Research methods in health promotion. Jossey-Bass; 2015.
11. Edberg M. Essentials of health behavior: essential public health. 3rd ed. Jones & Bartlett Learning; 2018.
12. Edelman CL, Kudzma EC Health promotion throughout the life span. Elsevier Health Sciences; 2021.
13. Ministry of Health (Saudi Arabia). Health education portal [Internet]. 2025 [cited 2026 Feb 17]. Available from: https://www.moh.gov.sa/awarenessplateform/Pages/default.aspx
14. Saudi Digital Library. Health sciences database collection [Internet]. 2025 [cited 2026 Feb 17]. Available from: https://sdl.edu.sa

School-Age Children and Adolescents

9

Learning Objectives

By the end of this chapter, students will be able to:

1. Describe the physical, cognitive, emotional, and social developmental characteristics of school-age children and adolescents, emphasizing how these stages influence health needs and behaviors.
2. Identify and analyze common health issues affecting school-age children and adolescents, including nutritional disorders, obesity, communicable diseases, injuries, and chronic conditions in Saudi Arabia and globally.
3. Examine the impact of mental health challenges—such as anxiety, depression, ADHD, and stress—on learning, behavior, and overall well-being, and outline appropriate nursing interventions and referral strategies.
4. Assess the influence of social determinants of health (e.g., family structure, socioeconomic status, culture, digital media, and environment) on child and adolescent health outcomes, particularly within the Saudi context.
5. Discuss the role of school health programs in promoting student well-being through preventive care, health screening, immunization, nutrition education, and mental health support.
6. Explain the multifaceted role of school nurses as clinicians, educators, advocates, and leaders in managing chronic illnesses, promoting health literacy, and fostering safe, supportive learning environments.
7. Design evidence-based health promotion and disease prevention programs for school settings, integrating interprofessional collaboration, parental engagement, and culturally appropriate health education strategies.
8. Evaluate the effectiveness of school health and adolescent programs using measurable indicators related to health status, academic performance, and psychosocial outcomes.

R. I. Ashgar, *Community Health Nursing: Principles, Practices, and Perspectives*,
https://doi.org/10.1007/978-3-032-30791-0_9

9. Utilize and appraise community resources to enhance care coordination and service accessibility for children and adolescents, emphasizing collaboration among schools, healthcare providers, and public health agencies.
10. Advocate for policies and initiatives that address emerging health challenges among Saudi youth, aligning with national health priorities and Vision 2030 goals for sustainable development and health equity.

Health Needs of School-Age Children

School-age children, typically defined as those between the ages of 6 and 12, represent a critical population segment characterized by unique health needs and developmental milestones. During this stage, children undergo significant physical, cognitive, and social transformations, necessitating a comprehensive approach to health promotion and disease prevention [1]. Physically, school-age children experience steady growth, requiring adequate nutrition to support their increasing energy needs. A balanced diet rich in essential nutrients, such as proteins, vitamins, and minerals, is crucial to foster optimal growth and development.

Health professionals must emphasize the importance of a nutritious diet while addressing the risks associated with obesity, which has become increasingly prevalent in this age group [2, 3]. Regular physical activity should be encouraged to promote cardiovascular health, strengthen muscles and bones, and maintain a healthy weight. Cognitively, this age group is marked by enhanced learning capabilities and the development of critical thinking skills. School environments play a pivotal role in shaping these cognitive abilities [4]. Consequently, community health nurses (CHNs) must collaborate with educators to create health-promoting school settings that support academic achievement and mental well-being. This collaboration can include programs focused on stress management, bullying prevention, and the promotion of a positive school climate. Socially, school-age children begin to form more complex relationships with peers and adults outside their immediate family. This development necessitates guidance in social skills and emotional intelligence. Community health initiatives can be designed to foster environments where children learn to communicate effectively, resolve conflicts, and build self-esteem [5].

Additionally, health education should cover the importance of hygiene, safety, and the prevention of communicable diseases, which are common concerns in school settings [3]. Furthermore, the health needs of school-age children are influenced by their family and community contexts. Socioeconomic factors, access to healthcare services, and cultural practices can significantly impact a child's health status. CHNs must consider these determinants when designing and implementing health interventions. By advocating for policies that improve access to healthcare and educational resources, nurses can help mitigate health disparities and promote equity [1].

The mental health of school-age children is another critical aspect of their overall health. Anxiety, depression, and attention-deficit disorders are increasingly recognized in this population, necessitating early identification and intervention [6, 7]. Health professionals should be trained to recognize the signs of mental health issues and collaborate with families and schools to provide appropriate support and resources. In summary, addressing the health needs of school-age children requires a multifaceted approach that encompasses physical, cognitive, social, and emotional dimensions. CHNs, educators, and families must work together to create supportive environments that promote healthy behaviors and prevent illness. Through targeted interventions and a focus on health education, school-age children can be equipped with the knowledge and skills necessary to lead healthy, fulfilling lives.

Adolescent Health Challenges

Adolescence is a critical transitional stage between childhood and adulthood, typically encompassing ages 12 to 19. It is characterized by significant biological changes (such as puberty), psychological changes (such as increasing independence), and social changes (such as evolving social relationships) [4, 5]. The World Health Organization (WHO) recognizes adolescence as a distinct life stage with unique vulnerabilities, requiring targeted interventions to support healthy development and prevent long-term health consequences [8].

During this stage, individuals face unique health challenges that require tailored interventions from community health nursing professionals. These challenges are influenced by genetic, behavioral, environmental, cultural, and socioeconomic factors. One of the primary concerns is mental health, as adolescents are particularly vulnerable to disorders such as depression, anxiety, and substance abuse [6]. These conditions can be exacerbated by factors such as peer pressure, academic stress, and social media influence. CHNs play a crucial role in early identification and intervention, providing education and resources to help adolescents navigate these challenges.

Physical health issues are also prevalent among adolescents, with obesity being a major concern due to its long-term health implications [9, 10]. The rise in sedentary lifestyles, coupled with poor dietary habits, has contributed to an increase in obesity rates among young people. CHNs can address this by promoting healthy eating and physical activity through school and community programs, aiming to instill lifelong healthy habits.

Sexual and reproductive health is another critical area of focus. Adolescents often lack accurate information and access to services, which can lead to unintended pregnancies and sexually transmitted infections (STIs) [4]. Comprehensive sex education and confidential health services are essential in empowering adolescents to make informed decisions about their sexual health. CHNs are instrumental in delivering these services and advocating for policies that support adolescent health needs.

Moreover, the influence of social determinants of health cannot be overlooked. Factors such as socioeconomic status, family dynamics, and access to healthcare significantly impact adolescent health outcomes [5]. CHNs must consider these determinants when designing and implementing interventions, ensuring they are culturally sensitive and accessible to all adolescents.

In addition to addressing individual health issues, community health nursing involves fostering environments that support healthy adolescent development. This includes creating safe spaces for adolescents to express themselves, promoting resilience, and building supportive networks involving families, schools, and communities. By adopting a holistic approach, CHNs can effectively address the multifaceted health challenges faced by adolescents, paving the way for healthier futures.

Health Challenges Among Saudi Children and Adolescents

Children and adolescents in Saudi Arabia represent a substantial and vital segment of the population [11]. As the Kingdom experiences rapid modernization and socioeconomic change, young people are increasingly exposed to a diverse set of health challenges that span physical, mental, emotional, and social domains. These challenges are influenced by lifestyle changes, urbanization, shifts in family dynamics, technological exposure, and evolving cultural norms.

Nutritional Disorders and Lifestyle Conditions

Childhood Obesity and Overweight [12, 13]

- Rates of childhood obesity in Saudi Arabia have reached alarming levels, particularly in urban areas.
- High-calorie diets, sugary beverages, limited physical activity, and sedentary screen-based entertainment contribute significantly.

Malnutrition and Micronutrient Deficiencies [6]

- In some rural regions, children face undernutrition or deficiencies in essential nutrients such as iron, vitamin D, and calcium.
- This can result in stunted growth, delayed cognitive development, and poor school performance.

Physical Inactivity [9, 10]

- Many children and adolescents do not meet recommended physical activity levels.

Mental and Emotional Health Issues

Rising Mental Health Concerns [7]

- Saudi children and adolescents increasingly face anxiety, depression, attention-deficit/hyperactivity disorder (ADHD), and emotional distress.
- Social isolation, academic pressure, bullying, and family problems are key contributors.

Impact of Digital and Social Media [14]

- Excessive screen time is associated with sleep disturbances, reduced physical activity, and increased feelings of loneliness.
- Cyberbullying and unrealistic social media standards negatively affect self-esteem, especially among adolescents.

Lack of Mental Health Resources

- Mental health services tailored to youth are limited in schools and primary care settings.
- Stigma and cultural barriers prevent many families from seeking professional help.

Risky Behaviors and Behavioral Disorders

Early Experimentation

- Adolescents may experiment with:
  - Tobacco and shisha
  - E-cigarettes
  - Caffeinated and energy drinks
- These behaviors are often driven by peer influence, curiosity, or lack of awareness about health risks [15].

Conduct and Behavioral Issues

- Behavioral challenges such as aggression, defiance, or social withdrawal can arise from neglect, inconsistent parenting, or academic struggles.

Reproductive and Pubertal Health Concerns

Limited Health Education

- Many young people lack knowledge about puberty, menstrual hygiene, fertility, and sexual health.

Early Puberty

- Increasing rates of early-onset puberty require appropriate education and emotional support.
- Misunderstanding bodily changes can lead to fear, shame, or misinformation among children and their peers.

Communicable and Vaccine-Preventable Diseases

Infectious Disease Risks

- Despite strong immunization programs, occasional outbreaks of measles, mumps, or influenza highlight the need for continued vigilance.

Chronic Diseases and Genetic Disorders

Asthma and Allergies

- Environmental factors such as dust storms, air pollution, and allergens contribute to high rates of asthma among Saudi youth [16].
- Poor disease management and inadequate parental awareness worsen outcomes.

Type 1 and Type 2 Diabetes

- Type 1 diabetes is increasingly common in Saudi children.
- Sedentary lifestyles and poor diets have led to rising cases of type 2 diabetes in adolescents [9].

Genetic Disorders

- Due to high consanguinity rates, genetic conditions such as:
  - Sickle cell disease,
  - Thalassemia, and
  - G6PD deficiency are more prevalent and require long-term care and family support.

Injury and Safety Concerns

Road Traffic Accidents

- Leading cause of death and disability among Saudi adolescents.
- Risk factors include lack of seatbelt use, speeding, and underage driving [17].

Home and School Injuries

- Burns, falls, and sports-related injuries are common.
- Lack of safety awareness and improper supervision contribute to preventable accidents.

Sleep and Academic Stress

Sleep Deprivation

- Late-night digital device use, caffeine consumption, and heavy homework loads disrupt sleep in children and teens.
- Sleep deficits impact memory, mood, academic performance, and immunity [1].

Educational Pressure

- Competitive school environments and high expectations lead to stress, anxiety, and sometimes school avoidance.

Developmental Delays and Learning Difficulties

- Early childhood developmental delays, including speech or motor issues, often go undiagnosed.
- Learning disabilities such as dyslexia or attention difficulties are underrecognized in schools, resulting in academic frustration and low self-esteem.

The health of Saudi children and adolescents is shaped by a complex interplay of biological, behavioral, environmental, cultural, and social factors. While notable progress has been made in healthcare access and public health campaigns, many challenges remain.

To address these concerns effectively, a multi-sectoral approach is essential, involving:

- Family and school engagement
- Community-based health promotion
- Mental and physical health service integration
- Policy development aligned with Vision 2030 goals

By investing in the well-being of children and adolescents today, Saudi Arabia ensures a healthier, more resilient population for tomorrow.

School Health Programs

School health programs are integral components of public health strategies aimed at fostering healthy behaviors among children and adolescents. These programs are designed to address the physical, emotional, and social health needs of students, thereby promoting optimal health and educational outcomes. The implementation of school health programs involves a multi-disciplinary approach, integrating efforts from healthcare professionals, educators, and community stakeholders [18].

The foundation of effective school health programs lies in their ability to provide comprehensive health services that cater to the diverse needs of the student population. This includes preventive services such as immunizations, screenings for vision, hearing, and dental health, as well as management of chronic conditions such as asthma and diabetes. By ensuring that students are healthy, these programs contribute to improved attendance and academic performance [5].

In addition to direct health services, school health programs play a crucial role in health education. Educating students about nutrition, physical activity, mental health, substance abuse, and sexual health empowers them to make informed choices and adopt healthier lifestyles. Health education curricula are tailored to be age-appropriate and culturally sensitive, facilitating effective communication and understanding among students from various backgrounds.

Mental health is a critical component of school health programs, given the increasing prevalence of mental health issues among young people. Schools provide a supportive environment where students can access counseling services and mental health resources. Early identification and intervention strategies are employed to address issues such as anxiety, depression, and bullying, thus fostering a safe and inclusive school climate.

Collaboration is key to the success of school health programs. Partnerships between schools, families, healthcare providers, and community organizations enhance the reach and effectiveness of health initiatives. These collaborations ensure that students receive continuous and coordinated care, both within and outside the school setting.

Moreover, school health programs are instrumental in addressing public health challenges such as obesity and infectious diseases. Through initiatives such as healthy school meals, physical education, and vaccination campaigns, schools contribute to the prevention and control of these conditions. The promotion of healthy eating and active living is emphasized, encouraging lifelong habits that reduce the risk of chronic diseases.

Evaluation and continuous improvement are essential to the sustainability of school health programs. Regular assessment of program outcomes helps identify areas for enhancement and ensures that the programs remain responsive to the evolving needs of the student population. Feedback from students, parents, and educators is invaluable in refining program strategies and interventions.

In conclusion, school health programs are vital in shaping the health and well-being of future generations. By addressing the holistic needs of students, these programs not only support academic achievement but also lay the groundwork for a healthier society. The commitment to fostering a supportive and health-promoting school environment reflects the broader goal of community health nursing to enhance the quality of life for all members of the community.

Role of School Nurses

School nurses play a pivotal role in the health and well-being of students, acting as a bridge between education and healthcare. Their responsibilities extend beyond mere first aid, encompassing a holistic approach to student health. School nurses are tasked with managing chronic conditions, preventing disease, and promoting health education among the school community [1, 4, 5].

In the context of chronic disease management, school nurses are crucial in monitoring students with conditions such as asthma, diabetes, and epilepsy. They ensure that these students receive their medication on time and that emergency protocols are in place and well understood by school staff. This proactive management not only safeguards the health of the students but also minimizes disruptions to their education.

Disease prevention is another critical aspect of the school nurse's role. This includes administering vaccines, conducting health screenings, and managing outbreaks of infectious diseases. School nurses are often the first to identify signs of contagious diseases, enabling swift action to prevent widespread transmission within the school. Their vigilance in monitoring and reporting health issues is essential in maintaining a safe and healthy school environment.

Health education is a fundamental component of the school nurse's duties. By educating students on topics such as nutrition, physical activity, mental health, and substance abuse, school nurses empower students to make informed health choices. They also provide guidance on sexual and reproductive health, helping students understand and navigate these complex issues responsibly.

In addition to direct health interventions, school nurses collaborate with teachers, parents, and community health resources to create a supportive network for students. They are advocates for student health, working to ensure that schools have the resources and policies necessary to support a healthy learning environment. This includes advocating for policies on healthy school meals, physical education, and mental health services.

School nurses also address the social determinants of health that affect students. They work with families to ensure that students have access to necessary health services, often connecting them with community resources for additional support. This holistic approach recognizes the impact of socioeconomic factors on health and seeks to mitigate these through targeted interventions.

Furthermore, school nurses are increasingly involved in addressing mental health issues within schools. They provide support and referrals for students experiencing mental health challenges, working closely with counselors and psychologists. By fostering an environment where mental health is prioritized, school nurses help reduce stigma and encourage students to seek help when needed.

In summary, the role of school nurses is multifaceted and integral to the educational experience. Their work ensures that students are healthy, safe, and ready to learn, contributing significantly to their academic success and overall well-being. School nurses are not just healthcare providers but also educators, advocates, and leaders in the school health community.

Community Resources

Community health nursing plays a pivotal role in enhancing the well-being of populations by leveraging community resources effectively. These resources encompass a wide array of services, programs, and materials that are accessible within the community to support health promotion, disease prevention, and healthcare delivery. The integration of community resources into nursing practice not only amplifies the reach and impact of health interventions but also fosters a collaborative environment that empowers individuals and communities alike [4].

Central to the utilization of community resources is the identification and assessment of available assets. This involves a comprehensive evaluation of both formal and informal resources, ranging from healthcare facilities, educational institutions, and government programs to community organizations, volunteer groups, and informal support networks. By mapping these resources, community health nurses can develop strategic partnerships and referrals that enhance service delivery and address the diverse needs of the population.

One of the critical aspects of integrating community resources is the establishment of strong interprofessional relationships. CHNs must collaborate with a multitude of stakeholders, including public health officials, social workers, educators, and community leaders, to create a cohesive network that supports holistic care. This collaboration not only facilitates the sharing of information and resources but also ensures that interventions are culturally and contextually relevant, thereby improving health outcomes.

Furthermore, CHNs play a crucial role in advocating for the development and enhancement of community resources. This involves identifying gaps in services, mobilizing community support, and engaging in policy advocacy to secure funding and resources necessary for the implementation of health programs. By acting as advocates, nurses contribute to the sustainability and resilience of community resources, ensuring their availability for future generations.

Education and capacity-building are also integral components of leveraging community resources. CHNs are tasked with educating individuals and groups about the availability and utilization of resources, empowering them to take an active role in managing their health. This involves conducting workshops, seminars, and outreach programs that raise awareness and build skills necessary for navigating the complex landscape of community resources.

In addition to education, CHNs must also focus on building the capacity of community organizations and groups. This includes providing training and support to enhance their ability to deliver services effectively and efficiently. By strengthening these entities, nurses help to create a robust network of resources that are capable of responding to the evolving health needs of the community. Ultimately, the successful integration of community resources into community health nursing practice requires a dynamic and adaptive approach. Nurses must remain attuned to changes within the community and continuously seek opportunities for collaboration and innovation. By doing so, they not only enhance the quality and accessibility of healthcare but also contribute to the overall health and well-being of the communities they serve.

References

1. Nies MA, McEwen M. Community/public health nursing: promoting the health of populations. 8th ed. Elsevier; 2023.
2. Centers for Disease Control and Prevention (CDC). School health guidelines to promote healthy eating and physical activity [Internet]. 2011 [cited 2026 Feb 17]. Available from: https://www.cdc.gov/mmwr/pdf/rr/rr6005.pdf

3. Chougule K, Halder A, Behere P, Chougule N. Prevalence, patterns and correlation of behavioral and emotional disorders in school-going children and adolescents: a cross-sectional study. Indian J Priv Psychiatry. 2024;18(1):19–21. https://doi.org/10.5005/jp-journals-10067-0153.
4. Stanhope M, Lancaster J. Public health nursing: population-centered health care in the community. 11th ed. Elsevier; 2024.
5. Seabert T, McKenzie J, Pinger R. An introduction to community and public health. 10th ed. Jones & Bartlett Learning; 2021.
6. Alsubaie A. Health concerns and health-risk behaviors among school-aged children in Saudi Arabia. J Fam Med Prim Care. 2025;14(3):825–31. https://doi.org/10.4103/jfmpc.jfmpc_1928_23.
7. Altwaijri Y, Kazdin AE, Al-Subaie A, Al-Habeeb A, Hyder S, Bilal L, et al. Lifetime prevalence and treatment of mental disorders in Saudi youth and adolescents. Sci Rep. 2023;13(1):6186. https://doi.org/10.1038/s41598-023-33005-5.
8. World Health Organization (WHO). Adolescent health [Internet]. 2025 [cited 2026 Feb 17]. Available from: https://www.who.int/health-topics/adolescent-health
9. Alasqah I, Mahmud I, East L, Usher K. Patterns of physical activity and dietary habits among adolescents in Saudi Arabia: a systematic review. Int J Health Sci. 2021;15(2):39–48.
10. Alasqah I, Mahmud I, East L, Alqarawi N, Usher K. Physical inactivity and its predictors among adolescents in Saudi Arabia: a cross-sectional comparison between cities with and without a Healthy Cities Program. Saudi Med J. 2021;42(8):886–94. https://doi.org/10.15537/smj.2021.42.8.20210310.
11. General Authority for Statistics (Saudi Arabia). Annual report 2024 [Internet]. 2024 [cited 2026 Feb 17]. Available from: https://www.stats.gov.sa/en/annual-report
12. Alshangiti A, Aldossary M, Abou-Hussein A, Aloufi W, El Dalatony M, Alomary S. Comorbidities of overweight and obesity associated risk factor in Saudi Arabia: a population-based analysis. Glob Health Action. 2025;18(1):1–7. https://doi.org/10.1080/16549716.2025.2477387.
13. Farsi DJ. Diet quality and physical activity and their association with BMI and dental caries among high school adolescents: a cross-sectional study. Children (Basel). 2024;11(11):1282. https://doi.org/10.3390/children11111282.
14. Faqihi F, Qutob R, Subh R, Aljathalin L, Alshalan L, Yati S, et al. Examining the effects of social media on mental health among adolescents in Saudi Arabia. Cureus. 2024;16(1):e53261. https://doi.org/10.7759/cureus.53261.
15. Alzahrani A. Teenage cigarettes smoking and the situation in Saudi Arabia in terms of prevalence, predicting and preventing factors: a narrative review. Eur J Med Health Sci. 2020;2(3). https://doi.org/10.24018/ejmed.2020.2.3.226
16. Alomary SA, Althagafi WA, Al Madani AJ, Adam IF, Elsherif OE, Al-Abdullaah AA, et al. The burden of asthma among children and adolescents in Saudi Arabia: a national cross-sectional survey. J Allergy Clin Immunol Glob. 2022;1(4):241–7. https://doi.org/10.1016/j.jacig.2022.07.006.
17. Babtain I, Almalki Y, Masud N, Asiri D. Unintentional injuries among young adolescents at a level-one trauma center in Saudi Arabia: a cross-sectional study. Cureus. 2023;15(3):e36645. https://doi.org/10.7759/cureus.36645.
18. Samad N, Bearne L, Noor F, Akter F, Parmar D. School-based healthy eating interventions for adolescents aged 10–19 years: an umbrella review. Int J Behav Nutr Phys Act. 2024;21:117. https://doi.org/10.1186/s12966-024-01668-6.

Check for updates

Client with Disabilities & Chronic Illness 10

Learning Objectives

By the end of this chapter, students will be able to:

1. Explain the multidimensional nature of disabilities, differentiating between physical, mental, and developmental impairments, and analyze how these conditions affect individuals' health, functioning, and participation in society.
2. Discuss the evolution from the medical model to the biopsychosocial model of disability and apply this framework to the holistic assessment and care of clients with disabilities in community settings.
3. Identify and evaluate the major chronic illnesses prevalent in Saudi Arabia—including diabetes, cardiovascular diseases, cancer, and chronic respiratory conditions—and describe their risk factors, prevention, and management strategies.
4. Develop individualized nursing care and self-management plans for clients living with chronic illnesses and disabilities, incorporating principles of patient education, empowerment, and interdisciplinary collaboration.
5. Describe the rehabilitation process and its components and assess the role of community health nurses in promoting recovery, independence, and quality of life.
6. Analyze the rehabilitation landscape in Saudi Arabia, including the roles of the Ministry of Health, Ministry of Human Resources and Social Development, and private and charitable organizations in providing inclusive care.
7. Utilize appropriate community resources and support networks to coordinate comprehensive services for clients and families, emphasizing culturally sensitive, person-centered care.
8. Demonstrate understanding of the policy frameworks and human rights principles governing care for persons with disabilities and chronic illnesses in Saudi

R. I. Ashgar, *Community Health Nursing: Principles, Practices, and Perspectives*,
https://doi.org/10.1007/978-3-032-30791-0_10

Arabia, including alignment with Vision 2030 and the UN Convention on the Rights of Persons with Disabilities.

9. Evaluate the role of advocacy and policy engagement in addressing barriers to accessibility, healthcare equity, and social inclusion for individuals with chronic conditions and disabilities.
10. Integrate concepts of rehabilitation, community support, and policy advocacy to design evidence-based, community-oriented interventions that promote inclusion, empowerment, and sustained health outcomes.

Understanding Disabilities

In community health nursing, a comprehensive understanding of disabilities is crucial for delivering effective care and support to individuals with diverse needs [1]. Disabilities encompass a wide range of physical, mental, sensory, and developmental impairments that may affect a person's ability to perform daily activities. These impairments can be congenital or acquired and may vary in severity, impacting individuals differently across their lifespan. Understanding the multifaceted nature of disabilities is essential for nurses to provide holistic care that addresses the physical, emotional, and social aspects of health.

The World Health Organization defines disability as an umbrella term covering impairments, activity limitations, and participation restrictions [2]. This definition highlights the importance of considering not only the medical aspects of disabilities but also the social and environmental factors that influence an individual's ability to participate fully in society. Community health nurses (CHNs) play a pivotal role in promoting inclusivity and advocating for the rights of individuals with disabilities by fostering environments that accommodate their unique needs [3,4].

Effective community health nursing requires a shift from a purely medical model of disability, which focuses on diagnosis and treatment, to a biopsychosocial model that considers the interplay between biological, psychological, and social factors [2]. This approach encourages nurses to view disabilities not merely as pathologies to be treated but as conditions that require comprehensive management strategies tailored to each individual's circumstances. By adopting this model, community health nurses can better support individuals in achieving optimal health and well-being.

Assessment is a critical component of understanding disabilities within the community health context. Nurses must conduct thorough evaluations to identify the specific needs and challenges faced by individuals with disabilities. This process involves gathering information about the individual's medical history, current health status, daily living skills, and social support systems. Additionally, nurses should assess the individual's environment to identify potential barriers to participation and access to services. Through this holistic assessment, nurses can develop personalized care plans that promote independence and enhance quality of life.

Education and empowerment are fundamental aspects of community health nursing for individuals with disabilities. Nurses have the responsibility to educate individuals and their families about the nature of their disabilities, available resources, and strategies for managing health effectively. Empowerment involves encouraging individuals to take an active role in their health care decisions and fostering self-advocacy skills. By providing education and support, nurses can help individuals with disabilities navigate the healthcare system and access necessary services.

Collaboration is another key element in understanding and addressing disabilities in community health nursing. Nurses must work closely with other healthcare professionals, community organizations, and policymakers to ensure that individuals with disabilities receive comprehensive and coordinated care. This collaborative approach enables the development of integrated care pathways that address the diverse needs of individuals with disabilities, from medical treatment to social services and community support.

In summary, understanding disabilities in the context of community health nursing involves recognizing the complex interplay of factors that affect individuals' health and well-being. By adopting a holistic, person-centered approach, community health nurses can provide effective care that empowers individuals with disabilities and promotes their full participation in society. Through assessment, education, empowerment, and collaboration, nurses are well-positioned to advocate for and support individuals with disabilities, ultimately contributing to healthier and more inclusive communities.

Chronic Illness Management

Chronic illness management within community health nursing focuses on the comprehensive care and support for individuals living with long-term health conditions [1]. These conditions often require ongoing medical attention and can significantly affect the quality of life and daily functioning of those afflicted. The role of CHNs is pivotal in providing holistic care that encompasses not only the physical needs but also the emotional, social, and psychological aspects of chronic illness [3].

Central to managing chronic illnesses in community settings is the development of personalized care plans that address the unique needs of each patient. This involves a detailed assessment of the individual's health status, lifestyle, and personal preferences. CHNs work collaboratively with patients, their families, and other healthcare professionals to establish goals that are realistic and achievable. These care plans are dynamic, necessitating regular reviews and adjustments in response to changes in the patient's condition or life circumstances.

Education is a cornerstone of chronic illness management. CHNs play a vital role in educating patients and their families about the nature of the illness, treatment options, and self-management strategies. Empowering patients with knowledge and skills to manage their conditions effectively can lead to improved health outcomes and enhance their autonomy. This educational process often includes teaching about medication management, nutrition, physical activity, and symptom monitoring.

Another critical aspect of managing chronic illnesses is the coordination of care across different healthcare settings. CHNs act as liaisons, ensuring seamless communication between primary care providers, specialists, and other healthcare services. This coordination is essential to prevent fragmentation of care and to ensure that patients receive comprehensive and continuous support.

Support groups and community resources are invaluable in chronic illness management. These resources provide patients with opportunities to connect with others facing similar challenges, fostering a sense of community and belonging. CHNs often facilitate access to these resources, helping patients to navigate available services and support networks.

Moreover, CHNs advocate for policy changes that improve access to care and resources for individuals with chronic illnesses. They work towards creating environments that support healthy living and reduce barriers to care, such as financial constraints or lack of transportation. Advocacy efforts are geared towards ensuring that healthcare systems are responsive to the needs of those with chronic conditions.

In managing chronic illnesses, the use of technology has become increasingly important. Telehealth services, electronic health records, and mobile health applications are tools that CHNs utilize to enhance patient care. These technologies enable better monitoring of health status, facilitate communication, and provide patients with easy access to health information and support. Ultimately, effective chronic illness management in community settings requires an integrative approach that combines medical care with social support and patient empowerment. CHNs are at the forefront of this effort, dedicated to improving the lives of individuals living with chronic conditions through compassionate and comprehensive care.

Prevalence in Saudi Arabia

Disabilities and chronic illnesses represent a growing public health concern in the Kingdom of Saudi Arabia, driven by demographic transitions, lifestyle changes, and improvements in healthcare delivery that have increased life expectancy [5,6].

Disability in Saudi Arabia

According to the General Authority for Statistics (GASTAT) 2023 disability survey [7]:

- 7.1% of the Saudi population is estimated to live with at least one type of disability.
- The most common disabilities include:
  - Mobility impairments (2.1%)
  - Visual impairments (1.5%)
  - Hearing impairments (0.8%)
  - Cognitive disabilities such as intellectual delays or memory loss (0.7%)
- Males are slightly more likely to report disabilities than females.
- Disability prevalence is higher among older adults and in rural or underserved regions.

- Geographic disparities exist, with higher prevalence rates in provinces with limited healthcare infrastructure.

Despite increasing awareness, many individuals with disabilities remain underserved due to limited accessibility, social stigma, and inadequate community-based rehabilitation services.

Chronic Illnesses

Chronic non-communicable diseases (NCDs) are the leading causes of morbidity and mortality in Saudi Arabia. The Ministry of Health and the World Health Organization report the following key statistics [8]:

- Diabetes Mellitus:
  - Affects over 18% of adults aged 20–79.
  - Type 2 diabetes is strongly linked to obesity and sedentary lifestyles.
  - Prevalence is projected to rise to 25% by 2045 if current trends continue.
- Cardiovascular Diseases (CVD):
  - Leading cause of death in the Kingdom.
  - Risk factors such as hypertension, smoking, dyslipidemia, and obesity are prevalent.
  - Hypertension affects approximately 15%–20% of adults.
- Obesity:
  - Approximately 59% of adults are overweight or obese, contributing to the development of diabetes, CVD, and musculoskeletal disorders.
  - Childhood obesity is also increasing, raising concerns for early-onset chronic illnesses.
- Cancer:
  - Cancer incidence is on the rise, with breast cancer being the most common among women and colorectal and liver cancer among men.
  - Late-stage diagnoses remain a challenge due to limited routine screening in some areas.
- Chronic Respiratory Diseases:
  - Conditions such as asthma and chronic obstructive pulmonary disease (COPD) affect a significant portion of the population.
  - Environmental factors like dust storms and tobacco use contribute to the burden.
- Chronic Kidney Disease (CKD):
  - Common among diabetic and hypertensive patients.
  - Over 17,000 patients are undergoing dialysis in Saudi Arabia, with increasing demand for organ transplantation

Rehabilitation Services

Rehabilitation services are integral to community health nursing, focusing on restoring individuals to their optimal functional capacity following illness or injury [9]. These services encompass a wide range of interventions designed to support physical, emotional, and social recovery, facilitating individuals' reintegration into their communities. Rehabilitation is a multidisciplinary approach, often involving collaboration among healthcare providers, patients, and their families to achieve the best possible outcomes [10].

The primary objective of rehabilitation services is to enhance quality of life by minimizing disabilities and promoting independence. This is achieved through personalized care plans that consider the unique needs and goals of each patient. Rehabilitation can occur in various settings, including hospitals, outpatient clinics, community centers, and even at home, depending on the individual's condition and requirements.

Physical rehabilitation focuses on improving mobility, strength, and coordination. It often involves physiotherapy exercises that help patients regain movement and function. Occupational therapy is another critical component, assisting individuals in relearning daily activities and adapting to new ways of performing tasks. Speech and language therapy may be necessary for those who have suffered a stroke or other conditions affecting communication abilities.

Emotional support is also a crucial aspect of rehabilitation services. Patients may experience anxiety, depression, or other psychological issues as they adjust to changes in their abilities and lifestyle. Counseling and mental health services provide the necessary support to address these challenges, helping individuals build resilience and coping strategies.

Social reintegration is facilitated through community-based programs that encourage participation in social activities and employment opportunities. These programs aim to reduce social isolation and promote a sense of belonging and purpose. Peer support groups can be particularly beneficial, offering a platform for individuals to share experiences and encouragement.

Family involvement is essential in the rehabilitation process. Educating family members about the patient's condition and recovery plan ensures they can provide appropriate support and encouragement. Family members may also need guidance on adapting the home environment to accommodate the patient's needs, such as installing mobility aids or modifying living spaces.

Technological advancements have significantly enhanced rehabilitation services, offering innovative tools and techniques to aid recovery. Tele-rehabilitation, for instance, allows patients to access therapy remotely, providing flexibility and convenience. Virtual reality and robotic-assisted therapies are emerging as effective methods for engaging patients in their rehabilitation programs, offering interactive and motivating experiences.

Despite these advancements, challenges remain in providing equitable access to rehabilitation services. Geographic, economic, and cultural barriers can limit availability, particularly in underserved communities. Addressing these disparities requires concerted efforts from policymakers, healthcare providers, and community organizations to ensure all individuals have the opportunity to benefit from rehabilitation services. In conclusion, rehabilitation services play a vital role in community health nursing, supporting individuals in their journey towards recovery and independence. By fostering a holistic approach that integrates physical, emotional, and social dimensions of health, these services contribute to the overall well-being and quality of life of patients. As the field continues to evolve, ongoing research and innovation will be crucial in overcoming existing challenges and enhancing the effectiveness of rehabilitation interventions.

Rehabilitation landscape in Saudi Arabia

The Kingdom of Saudi Arabia has made significant strides in expanding and institutionalizing rehabilitation services to meet the growing needs of individuals with disabilities and chronic illnesses. These services are provided through a collaborative network of governmental, private, and non-profit institutions, aligned with the country's national health strategy and Vision 2030 [11]. CHNs are instrumental in navigating these systems, referring clients, and ensuring continuity of care across healthcare settings.

National Framework and Policy Direction

A. Vision 2030 and Health Sector Transformation Program
Vision 2030 emphasizes inclusivity and equitable healthcare access for all population segments, including those with disabilities and chronic illnesses [12]. The Health Sector Transformation Program aims to:

- Enhance accessibility to specialized rehabilitation services.
- Develop community-based care models.
- Promote integrated care pathways from hospitals to home settings.
- Expand digital health and tele-rehabilitation programs.

B. Saudi Human Rights Commission & Disability Rights
Saudi Arabia ratified the UN Convention on the Rights of Persons with Disabilities in 2008. The Saudi Human Rights Commission, along with the Ministry of Human Resources and Social Development (MHRSD), ensures that people with disabilities have access to medical rehabilitation, education, employment, and social inclusion programs [11,13].

Governmental Organizations and Centers

A. Ministry of Health (MOH) Rehabilitation Services

The Ministry of Health operates several specialized rehabilitation hospitals and clinics across the Kingdom. Services include:

- Inpatient and outpatient rehabilitation for stroke, spinal cord injury, orthopedic trauma, and neurological conditions.
- Multidisciplinary teams including physiatrists, physical therapists, occupational therapists, speech therapists, and psychologists.

Key MOH facilities include:

- King Fahad Medical City – Rehabilitation Hospital (Riyadh)
- One of the most advanced centers, offering inpatient rehabilitation, prosthetics, and spinal cord injury programs.
- King Salman Rehabilitation Center
- Provides long-term and specialized rehabilitation for disabled individuals, including children and the elderly.
- Home Health Care Program – MOH
- Includes rehabilitation services for bedbound or mobility-impaired clients, with nurses and therapists conducting regular home visits.
- Diabetes Centers: A leading MOH facility specializing in the comprehensive management of diabetes, including education, medical treatment, and prevention of complications. These centers integrate rehabilitation services such as dietary counseling, foot care, and lifestyle coaching to support long-term disease control.

B. Ministry of Human Resources and Social Development (MHRSD)

This ministry plays a leading role in:

- Licensing disability care centers.
- Managing social rehabilitation centers and vocational training institutions for persons with disabilities.
- Offering monthly financial assistance, assistive devices, and transportation support.

Notable Centers:

- Comprehensive Rehabilitation Centers for Persons with Disabilities in each major city
- Al-Nour Institute for the Blind

C. Ministry of Education – Special Education and Support Services

The Ministry supports children with disabilities through:

- Inclusive education policies

- Special needs schools and support units for hearing, visual, and cognitive impairments
- School-based therapy programs in collaboration with MOH and MHRSD

Non-Governmental and Private Sector Services

A. Private Rehabilitation Hospitals and Clinics

The private sector plays an increasingly important role in:

- Offering specialized therapy, such as robotic rehabilitation and hydrotherapy.
- Reducing the burden on public hospitals.
- Providing services through health insurance for eligible clients.

B. Charitable and Community-Based Organizations

Several Saudi charities are actively involved in rehabilitation, including:

- King Salman Center for Disability Research
  Supports research, early screening, and policy development for disability-related issues.
- Disabled Children's Association (DCA)
  Operates centers that provide free therapeutic, educational, and rehabilitation services to children across the Kingdom.
- The Saudi Autistic Society
  Provide rehabilitation, family counseling, and educational services for individuals with autism spectrum disorder.
- SAUT – The Voice of Down Syndrome Society
  Offers comprehensive rehabilitation, family support, and educational programs for children with Down syndrome.

In conclusion, Saudi Arabia's rehabilitation landscape is rapidly evolving to meet the complex needs of individuals with disabilities and chronic diseases. The country's investment in specialized centers, policies, community-based programs, and technological innovations demonstrates a commitment to holistic, inclusive care. CHNs are vital in connecting clients with these resources, advocating for accessible services, and promoting rehabilitation as a right, not a privilege. As Vision 2030 unfolds, integrating rehabilitation into every layer of the healthcare system will ensure that all citizens, regardless of ability, are empowered to lead dignified, independent lives.

Community Support Networks

Community support networks play a pivotal role in the realm of community health nursing, providing essential frameworks that enhance the collective well-being of populations [1]. These networks consist of interconnected individuals and organizations that collaboratively work to address and fulfill the health needs of communities. By fostering relationships among community members, healthcare providers, and local organizations, these networks aim to create a supportive environment that promotes health and prevents disease [4].

The foundation of community support networks lies in the principles of mutual aid and collective responsibility. These networks operate under the premise that community members are both recipients and providers of support, thereby empowering individuals to take an active role in their health and well-being. This approach not only enhances individual health outcomes but also builds community resilience by leveraging local resources and knowledge.

One of the key components of successful community support networks is effective communication. Open lines of communication among network members facilitate the sharing of information, resources, and strategies that are critical for addressing health challenges. This communication is often facilitated by CHNs, who serve as liaisons between the healthcare system and the community. Their role is crucial in identifying community needs, coordinating resources, and advocating for policies that support community health objectives. Community support networks also emphasize the importance of collaboration among diverse stakeholders. By bringing together healthcare professionals, local government agencies, non-profit organizations, and community members, these networks create a comprehensive approach to health promotion. This collaboration ensures that interventions are culturally relevant, sustainable, and tailored to the specific needs of the community. Furthermore, these networks help to bridge gaps in healthcare access by providing support to underserved populations. They facilitate access to healthcare services, education, and resources, thereby reducing health disparities and promoting equity. For instance, community support networks may organize health fairs, vaccination drives, and educational workshops to increase health literacy and access to preventive services. In addition to addressing immediate health needs, community support networks play a significant role in building long-term community capacity. By fostering leadership skills among community members and encouraging participation in health-related decision-making, these networks empower individuals to advocate for their community's health needs. This empowerment is crucial for sustaining health improvements and ensuring that community voices are heard in policy discussions.

Overall, community support networks are integral to the practice of community health nursing. They provide a framework for collective action that enhances health outcomes and builds resilient communities. By fostering collaboration, communication, and empowerment, these networks create environments where individuals and communities can thrive. The role of CHNs in facilitating these networks is indispensable, as they bring together diverse stakeholders to work towards common health goals. Through their efforts, community support networks continue to be a cornerstone of effective community health interventions, promoting health equity and improving the quality of life for all community members.

Policy and Advocacy

Within the domain of community health nursing, the role of policy and advocacy is paramount in shaping the health landscape. This subchapter delves into the intricate relationships between policy formulation, advocacy efforts, and their impacts on community health outcomes. The dynamics of policy in health care are multifaceted, involving a complex interplay between government regulations, institutional policies, and community needs [6]. Nurses, as frontline health professionals, are uniquely positioned to influence health policy through advocacy, leveraging their firsthand experiences and insights into the health challenges faced by communities [3].

Policy in community health nursing is not merely about adherence to existing regulations but also involves active participation in shaping those policies to better serve public health goals. Policy development is a strategic process that requires comprehensive understanding and engagement with various stakeholders, including policymakers, community leaders, and healthcare providers. This engagement is essential to ensure that health policies are equitable, evidence-based, and responsive to the evolving needs of the population.

Advocacy in community health nursing extends beyond individual patient care to encompass broader public health issues. Nurses advocate for policies that promote health equity, access to care, and the social determinants of health. By doing so, they address the root causes of health disparities and work towards systemic change. Effective advocacy requires nurses to possess strong communication skills, a deep understanding of health policy, and the ability to collaborate across sectors.

The role of CHNs in advocacy is multifaceted. They serve as educators, raising awareness about health issues and influencing public perceptions. They act as collaborators, working with other healthcare professionals and community organizations to advance shared health objectives. Moreover, they are catalysts for change, mobilizing community resources and driving initiatives that lead to improved health outcomes.

One of the key strategies for effective advocacy is the use of data and evidence to support policy recommendations. CHNs must be adept at collecting and analyzing health data to identify trends and gaps in care. This evidence-based approach strengthens their advocacy efforts, providing a solid foundation for policy proposals and interventions. Furthermore, community health nurses must navigate the political landscape, understanding the power dynamics and decision-making processes that influence policy development. This requires political astuteness and the ability to build strategic alliances with policymakers and other influential figures. By engaging in the political process, nurses can contribute to the creation of policies that are not only effective but also sustainable and aligned with public health priorities.

In summary, the integration of policy and advocacy in community health nursing is essential for advancing health equity and improving population health. Through their advocacy efforts, CHNs play a critical role in shaping policies that reflect the needs and values of the communities they serve. Their contributions to policy development and implementation are vital in creating a health system that is responsive, equitable, and capable of addressing the complex health challenges of the 21st century.

References

1. Nies MA, McEwen M. *Community/public health nursing: promoting the health of populations*. 8th ed. Elsevier; 2023.
2. World Health Organization (WHO). International classification of functioning, disability and health (ICF) [Internet]. 2025 [cited 2026 Feb 17]. Available from: https://www.who.int/standards/classifications/international-classification-of-functioning-disability-and-health
3. Seabert T, McKenzie J, Pinger R. *An introduction to community and public health*. 10th ed. Jones & Bartlett Learning; 2021.
4. Stanhope M, Lancaster J. *Public health nursing: population-centered health care in the community*. 11th ed. Elsevier; 2024.
5. Alzahrani MS, Alharthi YS, Aljamal JK, Alarfaj AA, Vennu V, Noweir MD. 2023. National and regional rates of chronic diseases and all-cause mortality in Saudi Arabia: analysis of the 2018 household health survey data. Int J Environ Res Public Health. 20(7):5254 https://doi.org/10.3390/ijerph20075254
6. Hazazi A, Wilson. 2022. A. Noncommunicable diseases and health system responses in Saudi Arabia: focus on policies and strategies, a qualitative study. Health Res Policy Syst. 20:63 https://doi.org/10.1186/s12961-022-00872-9
7. General Authority for Statistics (Saudi Arabia). Disability statistics publication 2023 [Internet]. 2023 [cited 2026 Feb 17]. Available from: https://www.stats.gov.sa/en/statistics-tabs?tab=436312&category=123728
8. World Health Organization (WHO). Noncommunicable diseases [Internet]. 2025 [cited 2026 Feb 17]. Available from: https://www.who.int/health-topics/noncommunicable-diseases
9. Kuipers P. 2014. Empowerment in community-based rehabilitation and disability-inclusive development. Disabil CBR Incl Dev. 24(4):24 https://doi.org/10.5463/DCID.v24i4.274
10. Global Disability Summit. Global disability inclusion report [Internet]. 2025 [cited 2026 Feb 17]. Available from:https://www.globaldisabilitysummit.org/wp-content/uploads/2025/03/GIP03351-UNICEF-GDIR-Summary-v5-WEB-Accessible.pdf
11. Ministry of Human Resources and Social Development (Saudi Arabia). Empowering people with disabilities [Internet]. 2025 [cited 2026 Feb 17]. Available from: https://www.hrsd.gov.sa/en/empowering-people-special-needs
12. Vision 2030 (Saudi Arabia). Health sector transformation program [Internet]. 2025 [cited 2026 Feb 17]. Available from:https://www.vision2030.gov.sa/en/explore/programs/health-sector-transformation-program
13. Authority of People with Disability (Saudi Arabia). Overview of the rights of persons with disabilities in the Kingdom of Saudi Arabia [Internet]. [cited 2026 Feb 17]. Available from: https://apd.gov.sa/web/content/15711

11 Health Promotion and Risk Reduction

Learning Objectives

By the end of this chapter, students will be able to:

1. Explain the fundamental principles and philosophy of health promotion and their significance in empowering individuals, families, and communities to take greater control over their health determinants and outcomes.
2. Discuss the core components of health promotion, including participation, holism, equity, collaboration, and evidence-based practice, and analyze how these principles guide community health nursing interventions.
3. Identify and apply appropriate risk assessment tools and techniques—including epidemiological data analysis, health surveys, environmental scans, and risk stratification—to evaluate community health needs and priorities.
4. Utilize technological innovations such as electronic health records (EHRs), geographic information systems (GIS), and mobile health applications to enhance data-driven risk assessment and health promotion strategies.
5. Design and implement evidence-based intervention strategies that integrate health education, disease prevention, community engagement, advocacy, and interprofessional collaboration to address population health challenges.
6. Evaluate the effectiveness of community-based programs by applying participatory approaches, emphasizing prevention, promoting collaboration among stakeholders, and ensuring adaptability to evolving community needs.
7. Demonstrate understanding of monitoring and evaluation frameworks—including logic models and theories of change—to assess program outcomes, improve implementation processes, and ensure accountability in community health initiatives.
8. Apply theoretical frameworks such as Pender's Health Promotion Model, Health Belief Model, Transtheoretical Model, Social Cognitive Theory,

R. I. Ashgar, *Community Health Nursing: Principles, Practices, and Perspectives*,
https://doi.org/10.1007/978-3-032-30791-0_11

Ecological Model, and PRECEDE–PROCEED Model to the planning and evaluation of health promotion and risk reduction programs.
9. Critically analyze national and international health promotion success stories, including Saudi Arabia's Vision 2030 initiatives (e.g., Walk 30, Diabetes Prevention Program, Tobacco Control, and eHealth tools), to extract lessons applicable to nursing practice and policy development.
10. Synthesize knowledge of health promotion and risk reduction to formulate culturally competent, community-based nursing interventions that reduce health disparities and promote sustainable well-being across populations.

Principles of Health Promotion

Health promotion is a multifaceted approach aimed at enabling individuals and communities to increase control over their health and its determinants, thereby improving their overall health status [1]. This concept is rooted in the belief that health is a resource for everyday life, not merely the absence of disease. It encompasses a wide range of social and environmental interventions designed to benefit and protect individual health and quality of life by addressing and preventing the root causes of ill health, not just focusing on treatment and cure. The principles of health promotion are guided by several key tenets that form the basis for effective strategies and interventions [2].

First, health promotion is a participatory process. It involves individuals, families, communities, and populations actively engaging in efforts to improve their health. This participatory approach ensures that health promotion activities are relevant and culturally appropriate, and that they empower individuals and communities to take responsibility for their health [3]. Another fundamental principle is the focus on a holistic approach to health. Health promotion recognizes the complex interplay of various factors that influence health, including biological, psychological, social, and environmental determinants. By addressing these factors, health promotion seeks to improve not only physical health but also mental and social well-being. This comprehensive perspective is crucial in developing interventions that are effective in the long term [1]. Equity is also a core principle of health promotion. It emphasizes the need to reduce health disparities and ensure that all individuals have equal opportunities to achieve their full health potential. Health promotion strategies should aim to address the social determinants of health that contribute to inequities, such as poverty, education, and access to healthcare services [4]. In addition, health promotion is characterized by a settings-based approach. This involves implementing health promotion activities in the places where people live, work, learn, and play, such as schools, workplaces, and communities. By focusing on these settings, health promotion can create supportive environments that facilitate healthy choices and behaviors [4]. Furthermore, health promotion is an ongoing process that requires collaboration across sectors and disciplines. It involves partnerships between governments, health services, non-governmental organizations, and the private sector to create policies and environments that support health. This collaborative approach ensures that health promotion efforts are comprehensive and coordinated, maximizing their impact and sustainability [5]. Finally, health promotion is evidence-based. It relies on research and data to inform the development and implementation of interventions. This scientific basis ensures that health promotion strategies are effective and efficient, addressing the most pressing health issues and achieving the greatest possible impact [5].

In summary, the principles of health promotion provide a framework for developing and implementing strategies that improve health outcomes. By focusing on participation, holistic approaches, equity, settings, collaboration, and evidence-based practice, health promotion seeks to empower individuals and communities to take control of their health, ultimately leading to improved quality of life and well-being for all.

Risk Assessment Tools

Risk assessment tools play a pivotal role in community health nursing by enabling practitioners to systematically identify, evaluate, and address potential health risks within a community. These tools are essential for developing targeted interventions that promote health and prevent disease. One of the primary methods employed in risk assessment is the use of epidemiological data, which provides insights into the prevalence and incidence of diseases within a specific population. By analyzing this data, community health nurses can identify trends and patterns that may indicate emerging health threats [2].

In addition to epidemiological data, risk assessment tools often include health surveys and screenings that gather information on individual and community health behaviors, environmental factors, and genetic predispositions. These surveys can be conducted through questionnaires, interviews, or direct observation, and they provide valuable data that can be used to tailor health promotion strategies to the specific needs of the community [5,6]

Another critical component of risk assessment is the environmental scan, which involves the systematic examination of the physical, social, and economic factors that influence health outcomes. This includes assessing the availability and accessibility of healthcare services, the presence of environmental hazards, and the socioeconomic conditions that may impact health [5]. By understanding these factors, community health nurses (CHNs) can identify barriers to health and develop strategies to overcome them.

Risk stratification is another tool used in risk assessment, which involves categorizing individuals or groups based on their level of risk for developing certain health conditions. This process helps prioritize resources and interventions for those who are most at risk, ensuring that they receive the necessary support to improve their health outcomes. Risk stratification often utilizes algorithms and predictive models that incorporate multiple data points, such as age, medical history, and lifestyle factors, to determine an individual's risk level [5].

Furthermore, technology has become an integral part of risk assessment in community health nursing. Electronic health records (EHRs) and health information systems enable the efficient collection, storage, and analysis of health data, facilitating the identification of risk factors and the monitoring of health trends over time. The use of geographic information systems (GIS) also enhances risk assessment by providing spatial analysis of health data, allowing CHNs to visualize and address geographic disparities in health outcomes [6].

Effective risk assessment requires collaboration among various stakeholders, including healthcare providers, public health officials, and community members. By working together, these groups can share information, resources, and expertise to develop comprehensive risk assessment strategies that address the unique needs of the community. Additionally, engaging community members in the risk assessment process ensures that their perspectives and experiences are considered, leading to more culturally appropriate and acceptable interventions. In conclusion, risk assessment tools are indispensable in the field of community health nursing, providing a foundation for evidence-based practice. By systematically identifying and evaluating health risks, CHNs can develop targeted interventions that promote the health and well-being of the populations they serve. These tools not only enhance the ability to prevent disease but also empower communities to take an active role in managing their health.

Intervention Strategies

Intervention strategies in community health nursing are crucial to addressing the complex health needs of populations. These strategies involve a multifaceted approach that integrates evidence-based practices to enhance health outcomes across diverse communities. The primary objective is to empower individuals and groups to achieve optimal health through targeted actions and collaborations. One significant strategy is the implementation of health education programs tailored to the specific needs of the community [7]. Health education serves as a foundation for empowering individuals by increasing awareness and understanding of health issues. It involves disseminating information about disease prevention, healthy lifestyles, and available health resources. By tailoring educational content to the cultural and social contexts of the community, health professionals can ensure that the information is relevant and accessible.

Another critical strategy is the promotion of preventive health services. This involves identifying risk factors within the community and implementing screening programs to detect health issues early. Preventive services may include immunizations, screenings for chronic diseases, and health risk assessments. By focusing on prevention, CHNs can reduce the incidence of diseases and minimize the burden on healthcare systems.

Community engagement is also a vital component of intervention strategies. It entails collaborating with community leaders, organizations, and members to identify health priorities and develop appropriate interventions. Engaging the community fosters a sense of ownership and accountability, which is essential for the sustainability of health initiatives [3,8]. Through participatory approaches, CHNs can build trust and strengthen relationships, enhancing the effectiveness of interventions.

Moreover, advocacy plays a significant role in community health nursing interventions. Nurses advocate for policies and programs that address social determinants of health, such as poverty, education, and housing. By influencing policy changes and resource allocation, nurses can create an environment conducive to health improvement. Advocacy efforts also involve raising awareness about health disparities and promoting equity in healthcare access and quality.

Interprofessional collaboration is another cornerstone of effective intervention strategies. Community health nurses work alongside other healthcare professionals, social workers, educators, and policymakers to develop and implement comprehensive health plans. This collaborative approach ensures that interventions are holistic and address the multifactorial nature of health issues.

Finally, the evaluation of intervention outcomes is essential to determine the effectiveness of strategies and inform future practices. This involves collecting and analyzing data to assess the impact of interventions on health outcomes, community engagement, and resource utilization. Continuous evaluation allows for the refinement of strategies and the identification of best practices that can be replicated in other settings. In summary, intervention strategies in community health nursing are dynamic and require a comprehensive, collaborative approach to meet the diverse needs of populations. By focusing on education, prevention, community engagement, advocacy, collaboration, and evaluation, community health nurses can significantly contribute to the enhancement of public health and the reduction of health disparities.

Community-Based Programs

Community-based programs play a pivotal role in the realm of community health nursing, serving as essential mechanisms for addressing diverse health needs within populations. These programs are designed to leverage local resources, engage community members, and foster health-promoting environments through collaborative efforts. By focusing on the unique characteristics and requirements of the community, these initiatives aim to deliver tailored health interventions that are both effective and sustainable.

One of the fundamental aspects of community-based programs is their emphasis on participatory approaches [8,9]. This involves engaging community members in the planning, implementation, and evaluation stages of health interventions. Such engagement ensures that the programs are culturally relevant and aligned with the specific needs and values of the community. Moreover, it empowers individuals by giving them a voice in decisions that affect their health and well-being, thereby enhancing the likelihood of successful outcomes.

Another critical component of these programs is their focus on prevention and health promotion. Community-based initiatives often prioritize preventive measures over curative ones, recognizing that preventing illness and promoting healthy lifestyles can lead to more sustainable health improvements [10]. These programs may include educational campaigns on topics such as nutrition, physical activity, substance abuse prevention, and sexual health. By disseminating knowledge and fostering healthy behaviors, they contribute to the reduction of disease incidence and the enhancement of overall community health.

Collaboration is also a cornerstone of community-based programs. These initiatives often bring together a diverse array of stakeholders, including healthcare providers, local government agencies, non-profit organizations, and community leaders. Such partnerships are crucial for pooling resources, sharing expertise, and addressing the multifaceted determinants of health. Through collaborative efforts, community-based programs can tackle complex health issues that no single entity could address alone, such as social determinants of health, environmental factors, and access to care.

Furthermore, community-based programs are characterized by their adaptability and responsiveness to changing health needs. By maintaining a close connection with the community, these programs can quickly identify emerging health issues and adjust their strategies accordingly. This flexibility is particularly important in addressing public health emergencies or adapting to demographic shifts within the community.

Evaluation is an integral part of community-based programs, providing a mechanism for assessing their effectiveness and informing future efforts. By systematically collecting and analyzing data, program evaluators can determine whether the interventions are achieving their intended outcomes and identify areas for improvement. This process not only enhances accountability but also contributes to the evidence base for community health practices, guiding the development of more effective interventions. In summary, community-based programs are indispensable tools in the field of community health nursing. By fostering community engagement, emphasizing prevention, promoting collaboration, and maintaining adaptability, these initiatives address the complex health needs of populations in a holistic and sustainable manner. Through continuous evaluation and refinement, community-based programs can effectively contribute to the improvement of public health and the reduction of health disparities.

Monitoring and Evaluation

Monitoring and evaluation are critical components in the field of community health nursing, serving as mechanisms to ensure that health interventions are achieving their desired outcomes. These processes involve systematic assessment and continuous observation of health programs, aiming to enhance their efficiency, effectiveness, and sustainability [2,6]. The primary objective of monitoring is to track the progress of health initiatives, identifying any deviations from planned activities, and facilitating timely corrective actions. Evaluation, on the other hand, focuses on assessing the overall impact of health programs, determining their success in meeting objectives, and providing evidence-based recommendations for future improvements.

In community health nursing, monitoring involves the collection and analysis of data related to health service delivery and program implementation. This includes the use of indicators to measure inputs, processes, outputs, and outcomes. For instance, monitoring might track the number of community health workers trained, the frequency of health education sessions conducted, or the coverage of immunization programs. The data collected through monitoring are crucial for decision-making, enabling health managers to allocate resources efficiently and adjust strategies as needed.

Evaluation encompasses a broader scope, examining both the short-term and long-term effects of health interventions. It assesses the relevance, effectiveness, efficiency, impact, and sustainability of programs. Evaluative studies can be formative, summative, or developmental. Formative evaluation is conducted during the development or early implementation of a program to improve its design and performance. Summative evaluation occurs after program completion, focusing on its overall impact and outcomes. Developmental evaluation supports adaptive learning and innovation, particularly in complex or evolving health contexts.

The integration of monitoring and evaluation within community health nursing requires a structured framework, often guided by logic models or theories of change [4,11]. These tools help in clarifying the relationships between program activities and expected outcomes, establishing clear criteria for success and identifying key performance indicators. Effective monitoring and evaluation also depend on the active participation of stakeholders, including community members, health workers, and policymakers. Their involvement ensures that the evaluation process is inclusive, context-relevant, and aligned with community needs and priorities.

Challenges in monitoring and evaluation can arise from limited resources, insufficient data quality, and lack of technical capacity among health personnel. Addressing these challenges necessitates investments in training, capacity-building, and the development of robust data management systems. Furthermore, fostering a culture of learning and accountability within health organizations is essential for the continuous improvement of health services. In conclusion, monitoring and evaluation are indispensable for advancing community health nursing practice. They provide the evidence needed to guide decision-making, enhance program effectiveness, and ultimately improve health outcomes for communities. By systematically assessing the processes and impacts of health interventions, CHNs can contribute to more responsive, equitable, and sustainable health systems.

Theoretical Foundation for Health Promotion and Risk Reduction

The practice of health promotion and risk reduction in community health nursing is grounded in various theoretical frameworks that guide assessment, planning, intervention, and evaluation strategies. These theories provide a foundation for understanding health behaviors, predicting outcomes, and designing effective, evidence-based interventions tailored to individuals and populations [11,12].

Pender's Health Promotion Model (HPM)

Developed by Nola J. Pender, this model focuses on how individual characteristics and life experiences affect health behaviors. It assumes that people will commit to health-promoting behavior when they value the outcome and believe it is achievable [13].

Key Concepts

As shown in Fig. 11.1, HPM illustrates the key factors influencing health-promoting behaviors:

- Individual experiences (includes personal factors and prior behaviors)
- Behavior-specific cognitions and affect (includes perceived benefits of action, perceived barriers to action, perceived self-efficacy, activity-related affect, interpersonal influences, and situational influences).
- Behavioral outcomes (includes commitment to a plan of action, immediate competing demands and preferences, and health-promoting behavior)

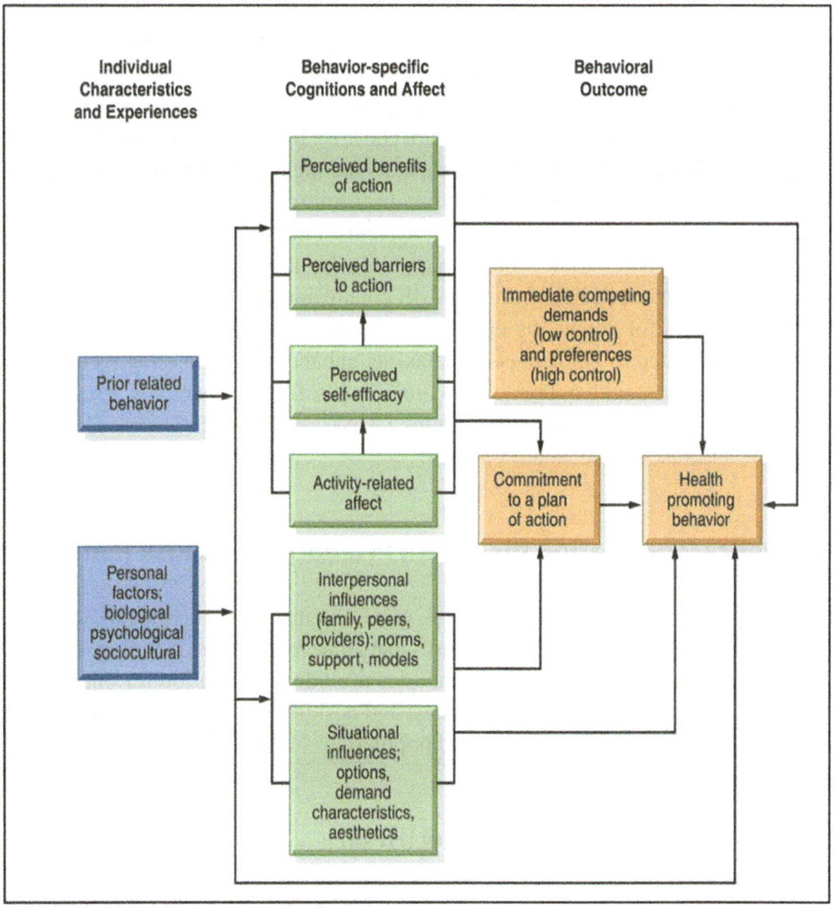

Fig. 11.1 Pender's Health Promotion Model (HPM)

Application in Practice

Used in designing school health programs, smoking cessation campaigns, and maternal health initiatives by addressing individual motivation and perceptions of health.

The Health Belief Model (HBM)

This model explains and predicts health behaviors by examining individual beliefs and attitudes toward illness and prevention [14,15].

Key Constructs

As demonstrated in Fig. 11.2, the HBM outlines factors influencing health decisions:

- Perceived susceptibility (belief about the chances of getting a disease)
- Perceived severity (belief about the seriousness of the condition)
- Perceived benefits (belief in the effectiveness of taking action)

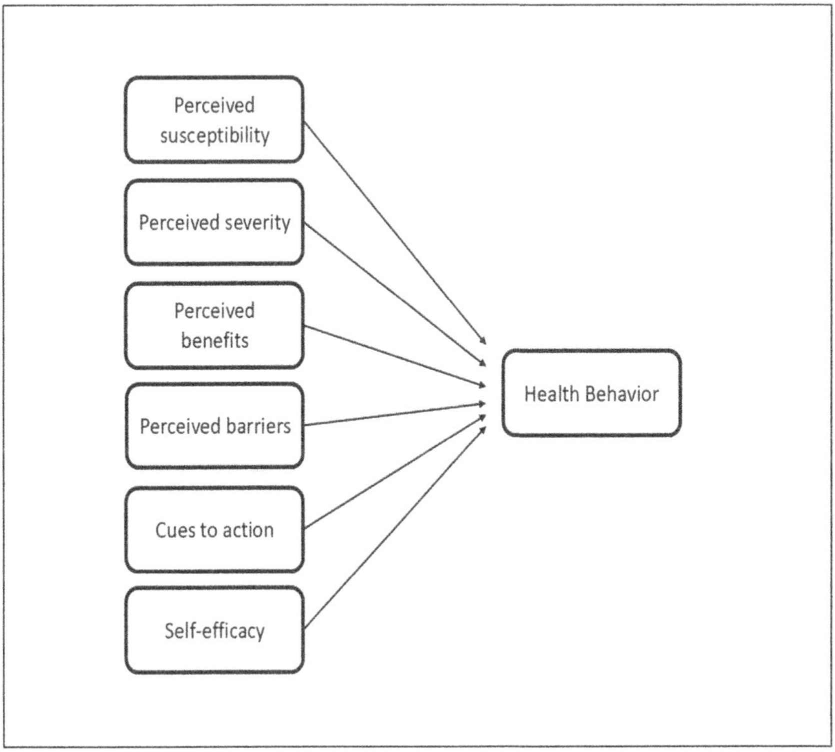

Fig. 11.2 Health Belief Model

- Perceived barriers (belief about the obstacles)
- Cues to action (triggers to prompt behavior)
- Self-efficacy (confidence in one's ability to take action)

Application in Practice

HBM is widely used in designing vaccination drives, breast cancer screening campaigns, and diabetes education by addressing perceptions that influence preventive actions.

Transtheoretical Model (Stages of Change Model)

Developed by Prochaska and DiClemente, this model views behavior change as a process occurring over time through five stages [12] see Fig. 11.3.

Stages

1. **Precontemplation** – No intention to change behavior.
2. **Contemplation** – Considering a change.
3. **Preparation** – Planning to take action.
4. **Action** – Actively modifying behavior.
5. **Maintenance** – Sustaining the new behavior.

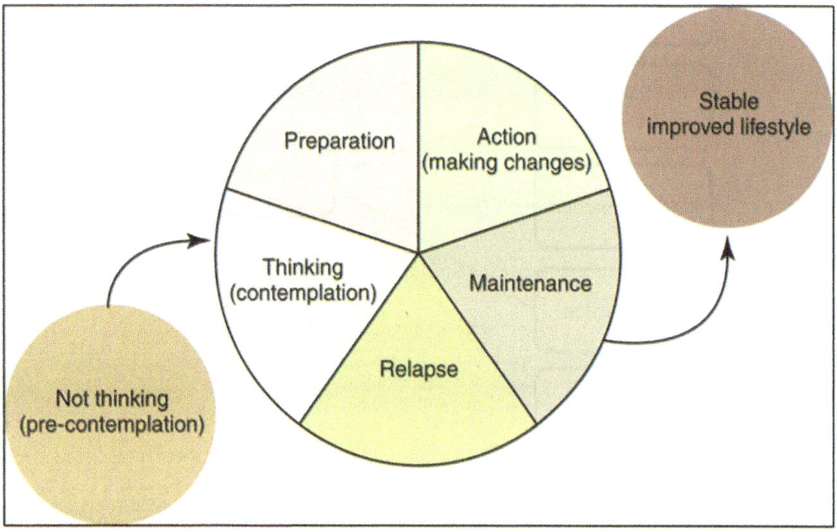

Fig. 11.3 The Transtheoretical Model

Application in Practice

CHNs use this model to tailor interventions, such as helping smokers quit or encouraging diabetic patients to adopt healthier eating habits, by aligning support with the individual's stage of change.

Social Cognitive Theory (SCT)

Formulated by Albert Bandura, SCT emphasizes the dynamic interaction between personal factors, behavior, and environmental influences (reciprocal determinism) [10,12]. Fig 11.4 depicts the components of Social Cognitive Theory.

Key Elements

- Observational learning (modeling)
- Reinforcement
- Self-efficacy
- Expectations
- Behavioral capability

Application

CHNs apply SCT to encourage healthy eating and physical activity by demonstrating behaviors and providing role models within the community.

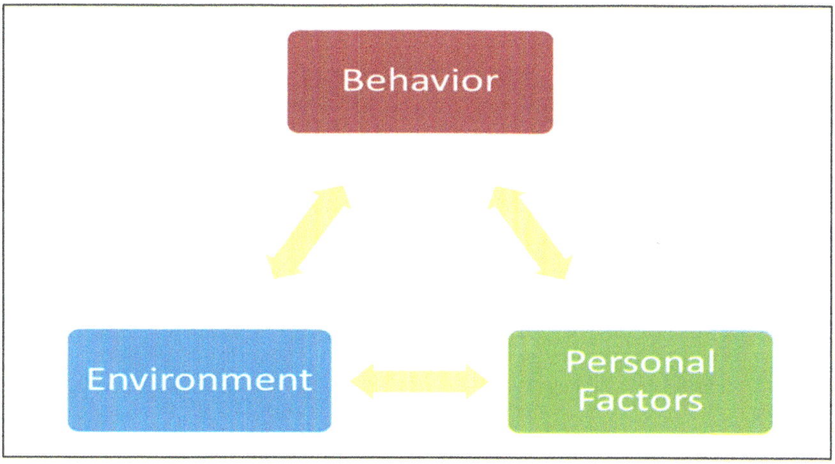

Fig. 11.4 Social Cognitive Theory

Ecological Model of Health Promotion

The Ecological Model of Health Promotion l looks at the multiple levels of influence on health behavior: individual, interpersonal, organizational, community, and policy levels [12]. The framework of the Ecological Model of Health Promotion is outlined in Fig. 11.5

Application

- Individual level: Health knowledge and attitudes
- Interpersonal: Family and peer support
- Organizational: School or workplace health policies
- Community: Access to health resources, cultural norms
- Policy: National laws and regulations (e.g., smoking bans, healthy food policies)

Application in Practice

Used in designing multi-level health programs like the Saudi Obesity Control Program, which integrates education, environmental changes, and legislative support.

PRECEDE-PROCEED Model

This planning model guides the development of health promotion programs by diagnosing health problems and designing interventions accordingly [1].

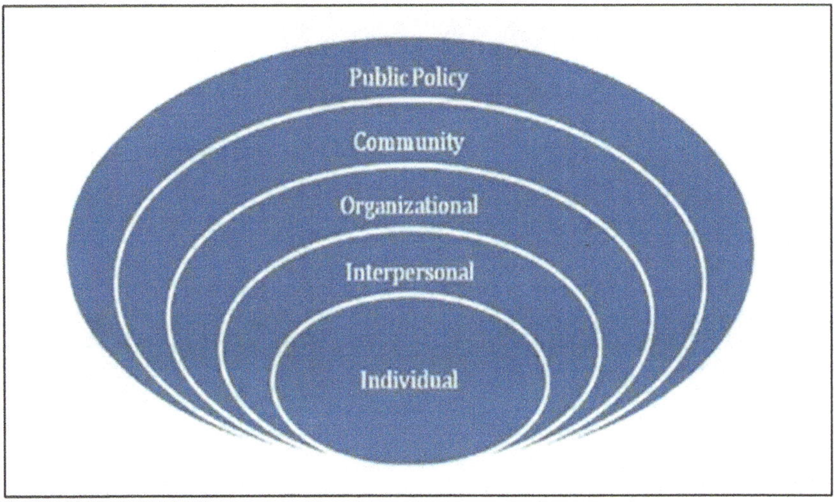

Fig. 11.5 Ecological Model of Health Promotion

Phases

- PRECEDE (Predisposing, Reinforcing, and Enabling Constructs in Educational Diagnosis and Evaluation)
- PROCEED (Policy, Regulatory, and Organizational Constructs in Educational and Environmental Development)

Application in Practice

Useful for needs assessments and structured planning in community health projects, such as school health services, maternal health education, and chronic disease management programs in primary care.

Summary of Application in Community Health Nursing

Model/Theory	Use in Practice
Pender's HPM	Motivating individuals to adopt healthier lifestyles
Health Belief Model	Designing health education to address personal beliefs and fears
Transtheoretical Model	Matching intervention strategies with an individual's readiness to change
Social Cognitive Theory	Using role models and enhancing confidence to encourage behavior change
Ecological Model	Developing holistic, multi-level interventions involving families, schools, and policy
PRECEDE-PROCEED Model	Systematic planning and evaluation of health programs

Success Stories and Examples

Saudi Arabia has witnessed a growing emphasis on proactive public health strategies aligned with its national transformation agenda—Vision 2030. This has led to the launch of several notable health promotion programs and risk reduction campaigns at the community level, driven by the Ministry of Health (MOH), nonprofit organizations, academic institutions, and private healthcare providers. Below are selected success stories that reflect effective implementation of health promotion and risk reduction in the Kingdom:

"Walk 30" Initiative

Objective:
To promote physical activity among the Saudi population, particularly targeting sedentary lifestyles—a key risk factor for noncommunicable diseases (NCDs).
Overview:
Launched by the Saudi Ministry of Health, the "Walk 30" campaign encourages individuals to walk for at least 30 minutes a day. It uses media campaigns, public events, and digital tracking tools to increase awareness and community engagement.

Impact:

- Significant public participation during events like World Walking Day and National Health Day.
- Incorporation of walking tracks in public parks and urban spaces.
- Notable reduction in self-reported sedentary behavior among participants.
- Alignment with MOH's "Quality of Life" goals under Vision 2030 [16].

National Diabetes Prevention and Control Program

Objective:
To address the rising prevalence of Type 2 Diabetes, which affects a substantial portion of the Saudi adult population.
Key Components:

- Free public screenings in malls, mosques, schools, and primary healthcare centers.
- Health education sessions on nutrition, physical activity, and medication adherence.
- Development of specialized Diabetes Centers within hospitals and primary health clusters.
- Use of mobile applications for glucose monitoring and appointment scheduling.

Outcomes:

- Improved early detection rates.
- Increased patient adherence to follow-up visits.
- Stronger integration of community nurses in chronic disease management teams [17].

Tobacco Control and Anti-Smoking Campaigns

Overview:
Saudi Arabia has enacted aggressive tobacco control policies alongside behavior-change campaigns to curb smoking, particularly among youth and young adults.
Strategies Implemented:

- Establishment of over 100 anti-smoking clinics across the Kingdom.
- Enforcement of smoking bans in public places, including airports, hospitals, and government facilities.
- Implementation of graphic warning labels and taxation on tobacco products.

Results:

- Decreased prevalence of smoking in targeted regions.
- Increased enrollment in smoking cessation programs.
- Notable success among adolescents where school-based interventions were applied [18].

National Breast Cancer Awareness Campaign

Goal:
To increase awareness and screening rates for breast cancer, particularly among women aged 40 and older.
Implementation:

- Mobile mammography units in remote and underserved areas.
- Media campaigns in collaboration with female influencers and local organizations.
- Educational seminars in universities, malls, and public places.

Impact:

- Significant rise in the number of early breast cancer detections.
- Increased community dialogue and reduction of stigma.
- Empowered female CHNs to lead local awareness sessions [19].

Health Education in Schools

Program Example

School Health Education— a school-based program implemented by the MOH in partnership with the Ministry of Education [20].

Objectives:

- Promote hygiene, mental health, and healthy eating habits among school-age children.
- Train teachers and school nurses as health ambassadors.
- Integrate health promotion into school curricula.

Achievements:

- Reduction in obesity and dental issues in participating schools.
- Improved student awareness of health risks and preventive behavior.
- Strengthened role of school health nurses in early identification of physical and emotional concerns.

eHealth and Mobile Apps for Risk Reduction

Saudi Arabia has invested in digital health tools to extend health education and self-management support [21].

Key Applications:

- Sehhaty App: Offers appointment booking, health records, virtual consultations, and fitness tracking.

- Tabaud and Tawakkalna Apps: Initially designed for COVID-19 tracking, later expanded to broader public health alerts and health status monitoring.
- Wasfaty: A digital prescription platform reducing medication errors and enhancing patient follow-up.

Impact:

- Expanded access to health services for remote and rural populations.
- Reduced healthcare system burden by empowering self-care.
- Strengthened risk communication during emergencies such as the COVID-19 pandemic.

In summary, these success stories demonstrate the effectiveness of community-level strategies, multisectoral partnerships, and culturally tailored interventions in achieving health promotion and risk reduction goals in Saudi Arabia. The role of CHNs has been central to these efforts, ensuring that education, engagement, and follow-up are adapted to local needs and values.

References

1. Murdaugh CL, Parsons MA, Pender NJ. Health promotion in nursing practice. 8th ed. Pearson; 2018.
2. Anderson ET, McFarlane J. Community as partner: theory and practice in nursing. 8th ed. Lippincott Williams & Wilkins; 2018.
3. Ashgar R. 2025. Community-based participatory research in cardiovascular disease prevention for middle-aged women: a systematic review. Heart Int. 19(1):12–19. https://doi.org/10.17925/HI.2025.19.1.1
4. Edelman CL, Kudzma EC. Health promotion throughout the life span. Elsevier Health Sciences; 2021.
5. DeMarco RF, Healey-Walsh J. Community & public health nursing: evidence for practice. 3rd ed. Lippincott Williams & Wilkins; 2020.
6. Caron RM, Noel K, Reed RN, Sibel J, Smith HJ. 2023. Health promotion, health protection, and disease prevention: challenges and opportunities in a dynamic landscape. AJPM Focus. 3(1):100167 https://doi.org/10.1016/j.focus.2023.100167
7. World Health Organization (WHO). Community engagement for quality health services [Internet]. 2025 [cited 2026 Feb 17]. Available from: https://www.who.int/teams/integrated-health-services/quality-of-care/community-engagement
8. Michener JL, Williams A, Oto-Kent D, Aguilar-Gaxiola S. 2025. Community engagement: a foundation for health equity and resilience. Am J Public Health. 115(Suppl):S104–S109. https://doi.org/10.2105/AJPH.2025.308029
9. Silberberg M, Cook J, Drescher C, McCloskey D. *Principles of community engagement*. 2nd ed. NIH Publication No. 11-7782. National Institutes of Health; 2011.
10. Salazar LF, Crosby RA, DiClemente RJ. Research methods in health promotion. Jossey-Bass; 2015.
11. Edberg M. Essentials of health behavior: essential public health. 3rd ed. Jones & Bartlett Learning; 2018.
12. Glanz K, Rimer BK, Viswanath K. Health behavior: theory, research, and practice. 6th ed. Wiley; 2024.
13. Pender NJ, Murdaugh CL, Parsons MA. Health promotion in nursing practice. 6th ed. Pearson; 2010.

14. Alyafei A, Easton-Carr R. The health belief model of behavior change. In: StatPearls [Internet]. 2024 [cited 2026 Feb 17]. Available from: https://www.ncbi.nlm.nih.gov/books/
15. Becker MH. 1974. editor. *The health belief model and personal health behavior*. C.B. Slack
16. Ministry of Health (Saudi Arabia). Walk 30 [Internet]. [cited 2026 Feb 17]. Available from: https://walking30.moh.gov.sa/
17. Saudi Health Council. Saudi diabetes clinical practice guidelines [Internet]. 2021 [cited 2026 Feb 17]. Available from: https://www.moh.gov.sa/Ministry/MediaCenter/Publications/Documents/Saudi-Diabetes-Clinical-Practice-Guidelines.pdf
18. Itumalla R, Aldhmadi B. 2020. Combating tobacco use in Saudi Arabia: a review of recent initiatives. East Mediterr Health J. 26(7):858–863. https://doi.org/10.26719/emhj.20.019
19. AlRajhi B, Aljadani FF, Almarwan SR, Alzahrani AA, Sindi MHM, Kano A, et al. 2023. Breast cancer awareness among women in Saudi Arabia: a systematic review. Breast Cancer (Dove Med Press). 15:913–924. https://doi.org/10.2147/BCTT.S426079
20. Ministry of Health (Saudi Arabia). School health education [Internet]. 2025 [cited 2026 Feb 17]. Available from: https://www.moh.gov.sa/Ministry/Projects/School-Health-Program/Pages/default.aspx
21. Masmali F, Miah S. 2021. Internet of things adoption for Saudi healthcare services. Asia Pac J Inf Syst. 31(3):113–130. https://doi.org/10.17705/1pais.13306

12 Disaster Management in the Community

Learning Objectives

By the end of this chapter, students will be able to:

1. Define and differentiate the major types of disasters—including natural, technological, complex emergencies, biological, and environmental degradation—and analyze their potential impacts on public health and community well-being.
2. Describe the phases of disaster management—prevention, preparedness, response, and recovery—and explain their interrelated roles in reducing vulnerability and enhancing community resilience.
3. Assess the role of community health nurses (CHNs) in each disaster management phase, emphasizing risk assessment, community education, emergency care, and long-term recovery interventions.
4. Apply principles of risk assessment and disaster preparedness planning to identify vulnerable populations, allocate resources effectively, and develop culturally appropriate community disaster response strategies.
5. Discuss evidence-based response strategies, including triage, search and rescue, emergency care, and mass casualty management, while maintaining ethical standards and cultural sensitivity in crisis situations.
6. Evaluate the processes of recovery and rehabilitation, including physical, psychological, and social dimensions, and propose nursing interventions that support individuals and communities in achieving post-disaster stability.
7. Analyze the concept of community resilience, identifying the social, economic, and environmental determinants that enhance a community's ability to prepare for, adapt to, and recover from disasters.
8. Examine the structure and functions of national disaster management systems in Saudi Arabia, including the roles of the Saudi Civil Defense, Ministry of Health, Saudi Red Crescent Authority, and local municipalities.

R. I. Ashgar, *Community Health Nursing: Principles, Practices, and Perspectives*,
https://doi.org/10.1007/978-3-032-30791-0_12

9. Identify the contributions of non-governmental and international organizations, such as the King Salman Humanitarian Aid and Relief Center (KSRelief), WHO, UNOCHA, and the GCC Disaster Risk Reduction Center, in disaster preparedness and humanitarian response.
10. Integrate principles of collaboration, communication, and evidence-based practice to develop a comprehensive disaster management plan that aligns with Saudi Vision 2030's goals for national resilience and health security.

Types of Disasters

Disasters, characterized by their potential to cause widespread harm and disruption, can be categorized into various types based on their origins and impacts. Understanding these types is crucial for effective disaster management and community health nursing [1]. Natural disasters are events caused by natural forces, such as earthquakes, hurricanes, floods, and tornadoes. These events often result in significant loss of life, property damage, and environmental destruction. Earthquakes, for instance, occur due to the movement of tectonic plates and can lead to catastrophic structural failures and tsunamis. Hurricanes, formed over warm ocean waters, bring strong winds and heavy rainfall, causing flooding and wind damage over vast areas.

Technological disasters, also known as human-made disasters, arise from human activities and technological failures. These include industrial accidents, chemical spills, and nuclear plant malfunctions. Such disasters often result from inadequate safety measures, equipment failure, or human error. The Bhopal Gas Tragedy and the Chernobyl nuclear disaster are sobering examples of technological disasters that had long-lasting health and environmental repercussions [2].

Complex emergencies, a type of disaster characterized by a breakdown of authority, often due to internal or external conflict, pose significant challenges for community health. These emergencies can lead to mass displacements, food shortages, and the collapse of health systems. The humanitarian crises in war-torn regions illustrate the devastating impacts of complex emergencies, where populations suffer from violence, malnutrition, and lack of access to essential health services [2].

Biological disasters involve the spread of diseases and biological agents, which can occur naturally or be human-induced. Epidemics and pandemics, such as the recent COVID-19 pandemic, fall under this category. These disasters highlight the importance of robust public health systems and preparedness plans to detect, respond to, and mitigate the impacts of infectious disease outbreaks [2].

Environmental degradation, although not a sudden disaster, can lead to situations that exacerbate the effects of other disaster types. Deforestation, climate change, and pollution contribute to the increased frequency and severity of natural disasters. They also pose long-term health risks, affecting air and water quality, and leading to increased incidence of respiratory and waterborne diseases.

In the context of community health nursing, understanding these types of disasters is essential for developing appropriate preparedness and response strategies.

Community health nurses (CHNs) play a pivotal role in disaster management, from conducting risk assessments and educating the public about disaster preparedness to providing emergency care and supporting recovery efforts [1, 3]. Their involvement is critical in enhancing community resilience and reducing the adverse health impacts of disasters. By comprehensively addressing the various types of disasters, CHNs can contribute significantly to safeguarding public health and promoting recovery in the aftermath of disastrous events.

Disaster Management Phases

Disaster management is a critical component in community health nursing, aimed at enhancing resilience and reducing vulnerability to public health emergencies. This involves a systematic approach to preventing, preparing for, responding to, and recovering from potential threats that may impact community health [4, 5]. The phases of disaster management are presented in Fig. 12.1. The process is rooted in a comprehensive understanding of the community's unique characteristics, resources, and needs.

Phase 1: Prevention

Prevention involves efforts to prevent disasters from occurring or to reduce their harmful effects. These measures often require significant investment but yield substantial long-term benefits in reduced disaster impacts. Key prevention strategies for disaster risk reduction encompass a combination of structural and non-structural approaches,

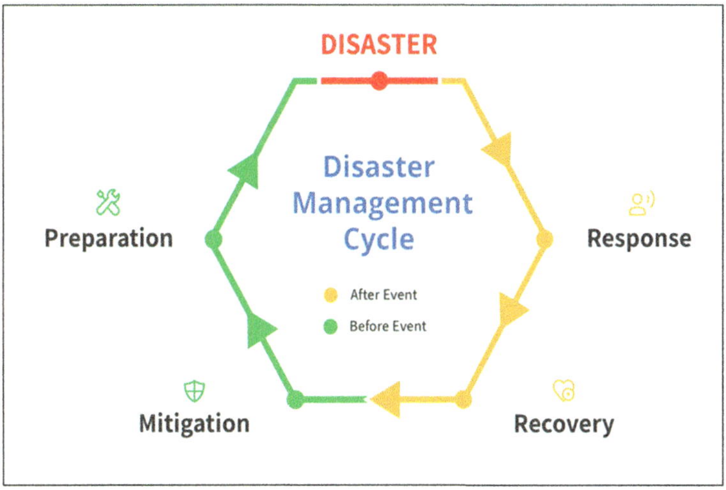

Fig. 12.1 Disaster management phases

environmental management, and thorough risk assessment [5]. These strategies aim to reduce the impact of hazards and enhance community resilience.

- **Structural measures** involve constructing physical defenses designed to withstand specific natural hazards. These include flood levees and seawalls to protect against water-related disasters, as well as earthquake-resistant buildings and infrastructure tailored to local geological risks. Such measures are critical in minimizing direct damage to lives and property during disaster events.
- **Non-structural measures** focus on policy and behavioral interventions that do not involve physical construction but significantly reduce vulnerability. These include land-use planning to avoid high-risk zones, enforcing building codes to ensure safe construction practices, establishing insurance programs to support post-disaster recovery, and implementing public education campaigns to raise awareness and preparedness within communities.
- **Environmental management** plays a vital role in prevention by maintaining or restoring natural ecosystems that act as protective buffers. For example, mangrove forests can reduce the impact of coastal storms and tidal surges, while reforestation can stabilize soil and prevent landslides in hilly areas. Preserving these natural systems is a cost-effective and sustainable approach to disaster prevention.
- **Risk assessment** is the foundation of effective prevention planning. It involves identifying potential hazards, analyzing vulnerabilities, and prioritizing areas and populations most at risk. This process enables authorities and planners to allocate resources efficiently and implement targeted measures that address the most critical threats. It requires collaboration with local, regional, and national public health agencies, as well as other stakeholders, to ensure a coordinated and effective response.

Phase 2: Preparation

While prevention targets the root causes of vulnerability, the preparation phase emphasizes the development of plans, resources, and capabilities to ensure an effective and timely response to disaster events [2, 5]. The development of a disaster management plan necessitates the establishment of clear objectives and priorities, which are informed by the risk assessment from the prevention phase. These objectives guide the allocation of resources and the implementation of interventions designed to mitigate risks. Importantly, the plan must be dynamic and adaptable, capable of evolving in response to new information or changing circumstances.

Training and education are integral to the preparation phase, ensuring that CHNs and other responders are equipped with the necessary skills and knowledge to effectively manage public health emergencies [6]. This includes regular drills and simulations that test the efficacy of the preparedness plan and identify areas for improvement. Community engagement is also vital, fostering a culture of readiness and ensuring that community members are informed participants in their own safety.

Communication is another essential component of the preparation phase. Effective communication strategies facilitate timely and accurate dissemination of information before, during, and after an emergency. This involves the use of multiple channels to reach diverse audiences and the development of messaging that is clear, concise, and culturally sensitive.

Partnerships play a pivotal role in the preparation phase, with CHNs often serving as liaisons between the community and various agencies. These partnerships enhance resource sharing and coordination, optimizing the overall response to public health threats. Collaborative efforts also extend to the development of policies and protocols that support preparedness activities and ensure compliance with regulatory requirements.

Evaluation and continuous improvement are fundamental to the preparation process. Regular review and updating of the plan are necessary to incorporate lessons learned from past incidents and to remain responsive to emerging threats. This iterative process involves the collection and analysis of data to assess the effectiveness of preparedness activities and to guide future planning efforts.

Phase 3: Response

The response phase of disaster management refers to the actions initiated immediately after the onset of a disaster [7]. Its primary objectives are to:

- Save human lives.
- Provide emergency medical care and basic needs.
- Prevent further injury or property damage.
- Stabilize the affected population and environment.

These activities are carried out under the guidance of established preparedness plans and are often coordinated by local, national, and international agencies, depending on the scale of the disaster.

Key Activities in the Response Phase

The response phase encompasses several urgent and coordinated actions, including but not limited to:

1. Search and Rescue Operations
Trained emergency personnel are deployed to locate and extricate victims trapped under debris, in flooded areas, or in other hazardous conditions. These operations are time-sensitive and rely on specialized equipment and techniques.

2. Triage and On-Site Medical Stabilization
Triage involves the rapid assessment and classification of victims based on the severity of their injuries and the urgency of medical intervention. On-site stabilization includes administering life-saving interventions before transporting patients to medical facilities.

3. Transportation of the Injured
Once stabilized, victims are transported to the nearest hospitals or emergency medical centers. This process requires coordination with ambulance services, traffic management authorities, and healthcare providers to ensure timely care.

4. Medical Treatment and Hospital Management
Hospitals and clinics play a crucial role in delivering emergency medical care. During mass casualty incidents, healthcare systems must activate surge protocols to accommodate increased patient volumes, manage resources efficiently, and maintain continuity of care.

5. Identification and Management of Deceased Individuals
In the aftermath of fatal disasters, the identification of deceased individuals, preservation of remains through refrigeration, and respectful handling of bodies become essential. This process also involves collaboration with forensic experts and communication with families.

6. Care of the Dead
Proper care of the dead includes documentation, cause-of-death verification, cultural and religious considerations, and the organization of burial or cremation services. This is essential for public health, legal processes, and providing closure to grieving families.

The effectiveness of the response phase depends on effective planning, rapid mobilization of resources, professional expertise, and strong coordination among stakeholders. Continuous evaluation and improvement of response protocols are necessary to enhance resilience and reduce vulnerability in future disaster events.

Phase 4: Recovery and Rehabilitation

Recovery and rehabilitation in disaster management is a critical phase aimed at restoring affected individuals, families, and communities to their pre-disaster conditions or better [2, 5]. This phase emphasizes a holistic approach that encompasses not only physical healing but also psychological and social reintegration. It is crucial to understand that recovery is a multifaceted journey that requires the concerted efforts of healthcare professionals, patients, and their families.

Recovery begins with a comprehensive assessment of the population's post-disaster needs, including physical injuries, mental health issues, displacement, loss of livelihood, and breakdown of essential services. CHNs play a central role in conducting these assessments and in identifying vulnerable individuals such as the elderly, people with disabilities, children, and those with chronic illnesses. This assessment informs the development of a personalized and community-wide recovery plan, which should be adaptive and evolving based on ongoing monitoring and feedback. CHNs are instrumental in coordinating multidisciplinary care teams, supporting health system recovery, and facilitating access to essential health and social services during this critical period [1, 3].

Rehabilitation is a key component of the recovery phase. It focuses on restoring functional abilities, promoting independence, and improving the quality of life for disaster-affected individuals. Interventions may include physical therapy, occupational therapy, speech therapy, and assistive devices, depending on the nature and extent of injuries or disabilities incurred during the disaster.

Beyond physical rehabilitation, the recovery process must address cognitive and emotional needs, especially in cases where trauma, grief, or loss has occurred. Mental health rehabilitation is often necessary and may involve psychological counseling, group therapy, or psychiatric care. CHNs are vital in facilitating these services, offering psychosocial support, and ensuring continuity of care across different stages of recovery.

The success of recovery and rehabilitation efforts is often measured by the community's ability to return to their pre-disaster level of functioning or better. Setting realistic goals and expectations is crucial for both affected communities and healthcare providers. In summary, recovery and rehabilitation in disaster management require a comprehensive, community-centered approach that integrates physical, psychological, and social elements. By fostering collaboration among healthcare providers, patients, and the community, nurses can help individuals achieve meaningful recovery and improve their quality of life.

Community Resilience

Community resilience is a multifaceted concept that plays a pivotal role in the field of community health nursing. It refers to the ability of a community to withstand, adapt to, and recover from adversity, whether it be natural disasters, economic downturns, or health crises [4, 5]. This resilience is not inherent; rather, it is cultivated through a combination of social, economic, and environmental factors that work together to support the community's health and well-being.

The foundation of community resilience lies in its social capital, which includes the networks, norms, and social trust that facilitate coordination and cooperation for mutual benefit. Social capital is critical in community health nursing as it fosters a sense of belonging and mutual support among community members. It enables communities to mobilize resources quickly and effectively in response to challenges. CHNs play a crucial role in building and maintaining social capital by promoting inclusive community networks and advocating for equitable access to resources.

Economic stability is another pillar of community resilience. Communities with diverse and robust economies are better equipped to handle economic shocks and recover more swiftly from disruptions. Economic resilience involves not only the availability of jobs and financial resources but also the equitable distribution of these resources across the community. CHNs can contribute to economic resilience by supporting programs that promote job training and education, which in turn enhance the community's overall health status.

Environmental factors also significantly impact community resilience. Healthy environments contribute to the physical and mental well-being of community members, reducing vulnerability to health threats. Environmental resilience involves sustainable practices that protect natural resources and mitigate the impact of environmental hazards. CHNs can advocate for policies and practices that promote environmental sustainability, such as clean air and water initiatives, which are essential for maintaining community health.

The integration of these elements creates a framework within which communities can develop resilience. However, fostering resilience requires a proactive approach that anticipates potential threats and prepares the community to respond effectively. This involves comprehensive planning and the development of strategies that are tailored to the specific needs and strengths of the community.

CHNs are uniquely positioned to lead these efforts due to their close relationships with community members and their understanding of the community's health dynamics [1]. They can facilitate resilience-building activities by engaging community stakeholders, identifying vulnerabilities, and developing targeted interventions. By promoting health education and preventative measures, community health nurses empower individuals and groups to take an active role in their health and resilience.

Furthermore, community resilience is enhanced through continuous learning and adaptation. Communities must be open to learning from past experiences and adapting their strategies to address new challenges [6]. CHNs, through their ongoing assessment and evaluation of community health programs, can provide valuable insights that drive this adaptive process. In conclusion, community resilience is a dynamic and ongoing process that requires the collective effort of individuals, organizations, and systems. Community health nursing, with its emphasis on holistic care and community involvement, is integral to fostering resilience. By addressing social, economic, and environmental determinants of health, CHNs can help build resilient communities capable of thriving in the face of adversity.

Disaster Management in Saudi Arabia

Effective disaster management requires coordinated efforts among a wide range of agencies and organizations at local, national, regional, and international levels. These entities play critical roles in disaster preparedness, response, recovery, and mitigation efforts. In the Kingdom of Saudi Arabia (KSA), disaster management is a national priority, guided by Vision 2030's goals for public health resilience and sustainable development [8].

Agencies and Organizations for Disaster Management

A. National Agencies in Saudi Arabia

1. Saudi Civil Defense (الدفاع المدني)

The General Directorate of Civil Defense is the central agency responsible for disaster response and emergency management in Saudi Arabia. Under the Ministry of Interior, it coordinates evacuation, rescue, firefighting, and hazard containment efforts during emergencies. Civil Defense is also involved in community education, risk assessment, and preparedness planning.

Key Functions:

- Emergency response coordination
- Search and rescue operations
- Hazard risk mapping and monitoring
- Public awareness campaigns
- Enforcement of safety regulations in the public and private sectors

2. Ministry of Health (MOH)

The Ministry of Health plays a critical role in ensuring health system readiness during disasters. It oversees emergency medical services (EMS), hospital preparedness, epidemic response, and the deployment of healthcare personnel [9].

Key Functions:

- Operating the Disaster and Emergency Management Center (DEMC)
- Coordinating mobile medical units and field hospitals
- Ensuring stockpiling of medical supplies and vaccines
- Conducting surveillance for outbreaks and bioterrorism threats

3. Saudi Red Crescent Authority (SRCA)

The SRCA is responsible for providing pre-hospital emergency medical care and ambulance services during disasters and mass casualty events. It also participates in disaster drills and public training in first aid.

Key Functions:

- Emergency medical transport and trauma care
- Mass casualty incident response
- First responder training
- Community disaster awareness programs

4. Ministry of Interior and Ministry of Defense

These ministries are critical during national emergencies, particularly for:

- Ensuring public security
- Supporting evacuation logistics
- Coordinating military and border operations in conflict-related disasters
- Managing high-risk mass gatherings such as Hajj and Umrah [10]

5. Local and Municipal Authorities

Municipalities across the Kingdom play a frontline role in disaster preparedness and recovery. Local health directorates, emergency committees, and public service sectors are responsible for:

- Assessing local vulnerabilities
- Enforcing building codes and environmental regulations
- Managing shelter and relief distribution
- Coordinating with hospitals and centers

B. Non-Governmental Organizations

1. King Salman Humanitarian Aid and Relief Center (KSRelief)

KSRelief supports both domestic and international humanitarian efforts. During disasters, it contributes to emergency logistics, food and water distribution, and shelter operations.

Key Contributions:

- Providing humanitarian aid during floods, earthquakes, and health crises
- Mobilizing volunteers and resources
- Supporting vulnerable populations in underserved regions

C. International Partnerships and Agencies

Saudi Arabia collaborates with international organizations to strengthen its disaster preparedness and response systems, particularly for health-related emergencies.

1. World Health Organization (WHO)

The WHO supports KSA through technical assistance in outbreak response, emergency preparedness planning, and capacity-building for health workers.

2. United Nations Office for the Coordination of Humanitarian Affairs (UNOCHA)

UNOCHA facilitates coordination between Saudi relief agencies and international partners, especially during cross-border emergencies and large-scale disasters.

3. Gulf Cooperation Council (GCC) Disaster Risk Reduction Center

The GCC Disaster Risk Reduction Center, based in Kuwait, promotes regional collaboration on early warning systems, emergency planning, and cross-border disaster response protocols among Gulf countries, including Saudi Arabia.

In conclusion, an effective disaster management system relies on the collective action of multiple agencies and organizations, each with distinct yet interconnected roles. In Saudi Arabia, national bodies such as the Civil Defense, Ministry of Health, and Saudi Red Crescent Authority lead coordinated disaster responses, supported by local municipalities, non-governmental organizations, and international partners. Community health nurses play a pivotal role in linking these efforts to the community level, ensuring that disaster management is inclusive, evidence-based, and grounded in public health principles. Strengthening inter-agency collaboration and capacity-building will be essential in achieving the national goals of resilience and health security outlined in Vision 2030.

References

1. Nies MA, McEwen M. Community/public health nursing: promoting the health of populations. 8th ed. Elsevier; 2023.
2. Coppola DP. Introduction to international disaster management. 4th ed. Elsevier Inc.; 2020.

3. Stanhope M, Lancaster J. Public health nursing: population-centered health care in the community. 11th ed. Elsevier; 2024.
4. McEntire DA. Disaster response and recovery: strategies and tactics for resilience. 3rd ed. Wiley; 2021.
5. Yokomatsu M, Hochrainer-Stigler S. Disaster risk reduction and resilience. Springer; 2020.
6. Bajow N, Mortelmans L, Maghraby N, Alatef Sultan S, Mani Z, Aloraifi S. Disaster health education framework for short and intermediate training in Saudi Arabia: a scoping review. Front Public Health. 2022;10:932597. https://doi.org/10.3389/fpubh.2022.932597.
7. Paton D, Johnston D. Disaster resilience: an integrated approach. 2nd ed. Charles C Thomas Publisher; 2017.
8. Mani Z, Sultan M, Plummer V, Goniewicz K. Navigating interoperability in disaster management: insights of current trends and challenges in Saudi Arabia. Int J Disaster Risk Sci. 2023;14:873–85. https://doi.org/10.1007/s13753-023-00528-4.
9. Ministry of Health (Saudi Arabia). Health emergencies: preparedness for health disasters [Internet]. 2025 [cited 2026 Feb 17]. Available from: https://www.moh.gov.sa/en/Ministry/Health-Emergencies-Preparedness-Disasters/Pages/default.aspx
10. Ridda I, Mansoor S, Briggs R, Gishe J, Aatmn D. Preparedness for mass gathering during Hajj and Umrah. Springer; 2021.

Check for updates

Environmental Health and Safety 13

Learning Objectives

By the end of this chapter, students will be able to:

1. Explain the concept and scope of environmental health within community health nursing, emphasizing the interrelationship between environmental, biological, chemical, physical, and social determinants of health.
2. Identify and analyze key environmental risk factors—including air and water pollution, hazardous chemicals, and biological agents—and evaluate their effects on population health and disease burden.
3. Discuss the roles and responsibilities of community health nurses (CHNs) in assessing, preventing, and managing environmental health risks through evidence-based interventions and community education.
4. Examine the principles of environmental health nursing, including prevention, precaution, advocacy, risk communication, sustainability, and interdisciplinary collaboration, and apply these principles to real-world practice scenarios.
5. Evaluate national and international policies and regulations governing environmental health and safety, including their implications for nursing practice, public health protection, and ethical responsibilities.
6. Design and implement effective community health initiatives that address environmental hazards, promote sustainable practices, and enhance community engagement in environmental decision-making.
7. Demonstrate understanding of sustainability practices in healthcare by integrating environmental, economic, and social dimensions into nursing interventions that promote long-term community well-being.
8. Apply environmental health principles to the Saudi Arabian context, particularly regarding air quality, water sanitation, waste management, climate change, and public health during mass gatherings such as Hajj and Umrah.

R. I. Ashgar, *Community Health Nursing: Principles, Practices, and Perspectives*,
https://doi.org/10.1007/978-3-032-30791-0_13

9. Analyze case studies that illustrate the application of environmental health principles in diverse community settings, and evaluate the outcomes of nursing interventions in addressing environmental and social determinants of health.
10. Synthesize knowledge of environmental health, sustainability, and community engagement to develop culturally competent, evidence-based, and policy-aligned strategies that enhance population safety and resilience against environmental risks.

Environmental Risk Factors

Environmental risk factors are critical components in understanding community health nursing due to their profound impact on public health. These factors encompass a wide range of elements including physical, chemical, biological, and social environments that can affect the health of individuals and communities. Recognizing and addressing these factors is essential for effective community health interventions and policies [1,2].

The physical environment includes natural and built environments where individuals live, work, and play. Natural environments comprise air, water, and soil quality, all of which can influence health outcomes [3]. For instance, air pollution from industrial emissions or vehicle exhausts can exacerbate respiratory conditions like asthma and chronic obstructive pulmonary disease (COPD) [4]. Similarly, contaminated water sources can lead to infectious diseases such as cholera and dysentery. Built environments, including housing, urban design, and transportation systems, also play a critical role. Poorly designed urban areas with inadequate green spaces and pedestrian pathways can lead to sedentary lifestyles, increasing the risk of obesity and cardiovascular diseases [5].

Chemical environmental factors involve exposure to hazardous substances in the air, water, and soil. These can include heavy metals like lead and mercury, pesticides used in agriculture, and industrial chemicals such as benzene. Chronic exposure to these substances can result in a range of health issues, from neurological disorders to cancers [3]. Community health nursing must focus on identifying these risks and advocating for policies that reduce exposure, such as stricter regulations on industrial emissions and safer agricultural practices.

Biological environmental factors refer to the presence of infectious agents in the environment. These include bacteria, viruses, and parasites that can cause diseases like influenza, tuberculosis, and malaria. The spread of these infectious agents can be exacerbated by factors such as overcrowding, poor sanitation, and inadequate healthcare infrastructure [3]. Community health nurses (CHNs) play a vital role in implementing vaccination programs, promoting hygiene practices, and educating communities about disease prevention to mitigate these risks.

Social environmental factors are equally significant and include socioeconomic status, education, and access to healthcare services. Communities with lower socioeconomic status often experience higher exposure to environmental hazards and have less access to healthcare resources. This disparity can lead to poorer health outcomes and increased vulnerability to environmental risks [5,6]. CHNs must work towards addressing these social determinants by advocating for equitable access to healthcare, improving health literacy, and supporting community empowerment initiatives.

In conclusion, environmental risk factors are diverse and interconnected, impacting community health in multifaceted ways. CHNs must adopt a holistic approach to identify, assess, and mitigate these risks. By doing so, nurses can contribute to creating healthier communities and reducing the burden of disease. This involves not only addressing immediate health concerns but also working towards long-term solutions that promote sustainable and equitable health outcomes for all community members.

Community Health Initiatives

Community health initiatives are critical components of public health strategies aimed at improving health outcomes and reducing health disparities within populations [2]. These initiatives encompass a wide range of programs and activities designed to address specific health concerns, promote healthy lifestyles, and enhance overall community well-being. A fundamental aspect of successful community health initiatives is the engagement and empowerment of community members, ensuring that programs are culturally sensitive and tailored to the unique needs and preferences of the community.

One of the primary objectives of community health initiatives is to increase access to healthcare services and resources. This can be achieved through the establishment of community health centers, mobile clinics, and outreach programs that provide preventive care, screenings, and health education. By improving access to healthcare, these initiatives help to identify and address health issues early, reducing the burden of disease and improving quality of life.

Education plays a pivotal role in community health initiatives. Health education programs are designed to increase awareness of health issues, promote healthy behaviors, and empower individuals to take control of their health. These programs often focus on topics such as nutrition, physical activity, chronic disease management, and substance abuse prevention. By providing individuals with the knowledge and skills necessary to make informed health decisions, community health initiatives can lead to lasting changes in health behaviors and outcomes.

Collaboration and partnership are essential for the success of community health initiatives. Partnerships between public health agencies, healthcare providers, community organizations, and local governments can enhance the reach and impact of health programs. These collaborations facilitate the sharing of resources, expertise, and best practices, enabling communities to implement comprehensive and coordinated health strategies.

Community health initiatives also emphasize the importance of addressing social determinants of health, such as housing, education, employment, and access to healthy foods. By tackling these underlying factors, initiatives can create environments that support healthy living and reduce health inequities. Strategies may include advocating for policies that promote affordable housing, improving access to quality education, and supporting local food systems to ensure the availability of nutritious foods.

Evaluation and assessment are critical components of community health initiatives, allowing stakeholders to measure the effectiveness of programs and make data-driven decisions. By collecting and analyzing data on health outcomes, program participation, and community feedback, initiatives can identify areas for improvement and demonstrate their impact on community health.

In summary, community health initiatives are vital for promoting health equity and improving population health. Through increased access to healthcare, health education, collaboration, and a focus on social determinants, these initiatives can create healthier communities and enhance the quality of life for individuals. By continuously evaluating and refining their approaches, community health initiatives can adapt to changing needs and ensure their long-term success.

Policies and Regulations

In the realm of community health nursing, policies and regulations serve as the cornerstone for ensuring that healthcare practices are equitable, effective, and aligned with public health goals. These frameworks are designed to guide nurses in delivering care that is not only consistent with professional standards but also responsive to the needs of diverse populations. At the heart of these regulations is the objective to safeguard public health while fostering an environment that supports the well-being and dignity of all individuals [1].

Central to the development of these policies are governmental and non-governmental organizations that collaborate to establish guidelines that reflect the latest scientific advancements and ethical considerations. The policies are often influenced by epidemiological data, which provides insights into health trends and informs preventative strategies. Regulations are periodically reviewed and updated to incorporate new findings and address emerging health challenges, ensuring that community health nursing remains adaptable and forward-thinking.

One of the primary roles of policies in community health nursing is to standardize care across different settings. This standardization helps in reducing disparities in health services and outcomes, particularly among vulnerable populations [7]. For instance, policies may dictate specific interventions for managing chronic diseases or outline protocols for immunization programs. By adhering to these guidelines, CHNs can deliver care that minimizes risks and enhances patient outcomes.

Moreover, policies and regulations play a crucial role in defining the scope of practice for community health nurses. They outline the responsibilities and limitations within which nurses operate, thus providing a clear framework that supports professional practice. This clarity is essential not only for maintaining the quality of care but also for protecting nurses from potential legal liabilities. Additionally, these regulations often include provisions for continuing education and professional development, ensuring that nurses remain competent and informed about the latest practices.

In the context of health promotion and disease prevention, policies are instrumental in shaping initiatives that target specific health issues. For example, regulations may support programs aimed at reducing tobacco use, promoting physical activity, or improving nutritional standards in schools. These initiatives are typically grounded in evidence-based practices and require the active involvement of CHNs to implement and evaluate their effectiveness.

Furthermore, ethical considerations are a vital component of the regulatory framework in community health nursing. Policies are designed to uphold principles such as confidentiality, informed consent, and cultural sensitivity. These ethical guidelines ensure that nurses respect the rights and autonomy of individuals while providing care that is empathetic and respectful of cultural differences.

In summary, policies and regulations in community health nursing are essential for guiding practice, ensuring quality care, and protecting both patients and healthcare providers. They provide a structured approach to addressing public health challenges and contribute to the overall improvement of health outcomes in communities. As the field of community health continues to evolve, these regulatory frameworks will remain pivotal in shaping the future of nursing practice.

Sustainability Practices

In the realm of community health nursing, sustainability practices are increasingly acknowledged as integral to fostering long-term health and well-being. These practices not only aim to address immediate health needs but also seek to ensure the enduring viability of health systems and resources for future generations. Central to this approach is the recognition of the intricate interplay between environmental, economic, and social factors in shaping health outcomes [5].

CHNs play a pivotal role in advancing sustainability by integrating eco-friendly strategies into their practice. This involves advocating for and implementing measures that minimize environmental impact, such as reducing waste, promoting energy efficiency, and supporting the use of sustainable materials and technologies. By doing so, nurses contribute to the reduction of the healthcare sector's carbon footprint, thereby aligning with broader environmental sustainability goals.

Economic sustainability is another critical dimension that CHNs must consider. This entails ensuring that health interventions are cost-effective and accessible, particularly for underserved populations. Nurses are often at the forefront of efforts to optimize resource allocation, advocating for equitable distribution of healthcare resources and services. This may involve collaborating with community organizations, policymakers, and other stakeholders to develop and implement policies that support sustainable healthcare financing and delivery models.

Social sustainability, which encompasses the promotion of health equity and social justice, is also a cornerstone of sustainable community health nursing practice. Nurses are tasked with addressing social determinants of health, such as education, employment, and housing, which significantly influence health outcomes. By engaging with communities and fostering partnerships, nurses can help build resilient communities that are better equipped to withstand health challenges and disparities.

Education and advocacy are key components of sustainability practices in community health nursing [7]. Nurses must be equipped with the knowledge and skills necessary to educate communities about sustainable health practices and the importance of maintaining healthy environments. This involves not only imparting information but also empowering individuals and communities to take an active role in their health and well-being.

Moreover, CHNs can advocate for policies and practices that support sustainable health systems. This includes participating in health policy development, engaging in research to identify effective sustainability interventions, and collaborating with interdisciplinary teams to implement evidence-based practices. Through these efforts, nurses can help shape a healthcare landscape that prioritizes sustainability and resilience.

In conclusion, sustainability practices in community health nursing are essential for ensuring the long-term health and well-being of populations. By addressing environmental, economic, and social dimensions of sustainability, nurses can contribute to the creation of health systems that are not only effective and efficient but also equitable and resilient. As advocates, educators, and practitioners, CHNs are uniquely positioned to lead the charge towards a more sustainable future in healthcare.

Principles of Environmental Health Nursing

Environmental health nursing is a specialized area within community health nursing that focuses on identifying, preventing, and managing health issues arising from environmental factors. It emphasizes the critical relationship between human health and environmental conditions, including air, water, soil quality, and the built environment [8]. Nurses practicing in this field work to safeguard public health by assessing environmental risks, promoting sustainable practices, and advocating for policy changes to reduce exposure to environmental hazards.

Core Principles of Environmental Health Nursing

1. Prevention and Precaution

Prevention is a foundational principle of environmental health nursing. Nurses aim to reduce or eliminate environmental risks before they cause harm. This involves early identification of potential environmental threats, implementing interventions, and promoting policies that mitigate risk. The precautionary principle further guides practice by recommending action even when scientific certainty about harm is lacking, especially when vulnerable populations like children or the elderly are at risk.

2. Assessment of Environmental Hazards
Environmental health nurses perform comprehensive assessments to identify potential hazards in homes, workplaces, schools, and communities. This includes evaluating air and water quality, toxic exposures, noise pollution, radiation, and housing conditions. Tools such as environmental history taking, risk mapping, and exposure pathway analysis help in understanding the links between environmental exposures and health outcomes.

3. Health Education and Risk Communication
Effective communication is vital in empowering individuals and communities to make informed decisions about their environment. Environmental health nurses educate communities on safe practices, such as proper waste disposal, pesticide use, water purification, and lead paint removal. They also communicate risks in an accessible, culturally sensitive manner, tailoring messages to diverse populations and literacy levels.

4. Advocacy and Policy Engagement
Environmental health nurses play an important role as advocates for healthier environments. This includes participating in policy development, supporting legislation that promotes environmental justice, and collaborating with interdisciplinary teams to influence local, national, and global environmental health agendas. Advocacy efforts often focus on protecting marginalized or disadvantaged populations that are disproportionately affected by environmental hazards.

5. Community Participation and Empowerment
Community engagement is central to environmental health nursing. Nurses collaborate with community members, leaders, and organizations to identify concerns, set priorities, and co-develop interventions. Empowering communities fosters ownership of health initiatives and leads to sustainable environmental improvements.

6. Cultural and Ethical Sensitivity
Environmental health interventions must be ethically sound and culturally appropriate. Nurses must respect traditional practices while promoting evidence-based solutions to environmental problems. Ethical considerations include the right to a clean and safe environment, equitable access to resources, and transparency in communicating risks.

7. Sustainability and Stewardship
Nurses contribute to environmental sustainability by promoting eco-friendly practices in healthcare settings and the community. This includes reducing healthcare waste, encouraging the use of renewable resources, supporting green infrastructure, and educating others about sustainable living. Environmental stewardship reflects a commitment to future generations.

8. Interdisciplinary Collaboration
Environmental health nursing requires collaboration across sectors, including public health, environmental sciences, urban planning, toxicology, and engineering. Working with professionals from diverse disciplines enhances the effectiveness of interventions and fosters holistic approaches to environmental health issues.

Competencies of Environmental Health Nurses

Key competencies for environmental health nursing include:

- Conducting environmental health assessments
- Understanding toxicology and exposure science
- Applying epidemiological methods
- Communicating risks effectively
- Advocating for vulnerable populations
- Collaborating with multidisciplinary teams
- Implementing and evaluating environmental interventions [1]

Application of Environmental Health Principles in Saudi Arabia

Saudi Arabia's unique environmental and socio-economic context demands tailored applications of environmental health nursing principles. The Kingdom is characterized by arid climates, rapid urbanization, a growing industrial base, population concentration in urban centers, and periodic mass gatherings such as Hajj and Umrah. These factors contribute to a complex web of environmental health challenges that necessitate proactive, culturally sensitive, and evidence-based nursing interventions [9,10]. The following domains illustrate how environmental health principles are operationalized within the Saudi context.

Air Quality and Respiratory Health

Major cities such as Riyadh, Jeddah, and Dammam face air pollution challenges due to industrial emissions, vehicle exhaust, and frequent dust storms. Nurses play a pivotal role in educating the public about indoor air purification, asthma management, and minimizing outdoor exposure during high pollution events.

Water Sanitation and Safety

Access to clean water is vital. While Saudi Arabia has advanced desalination infrastructure, issues like pipeline contamination and inadequate water storage practices in rural areas can pose health risks. Nurses conduct water safety education and can collaborate with health inspectors to monitor water quality in homes and public institutions.

Waste Management

Inadequate waste disposal, especially in informal settlements or during mass gatherings like Hajj, increases the risk of vector-borne diseases and environmental degradation.

Nurses contribute to waste management campaigns, particularly regarding medical waste and community-level hygiene practices.

Climate Change and Public Health

With increasing temperatures and extreme weather events, climate-sensitive health issues are emerging. Environmental health nurses support heat-related illness prevention campaigns, encourage hydration awareness, and promote green health initiatives as part of national climate adaptation efforts.

Public Health During Mass Gatherings (Hajj and Umrah)

Mass gatherings in Mecca and Medina attract millions of pilgrims each year, placing significant strain on environmental infrastructure, sanitation systems, and public health services. Environmental health nurses play a critical role during these events by monitoring sanitation conditions, evaluating food and water safety, and ensuring hygienic standards in pilgrim accommodations. They also participate in intersectoral emergency preparedness drills and lead culturally and linguistically appropriate health education campaigns. Furthermore, nurses contribute to infectious disease surveillance and support the early detection and containment of outbreaks—particularly those related to environmental transmission pathways, such as cholera and Middle East Respiratory Syndrome Coronavirus (MERS-CoV).

Case Studies

Case studies serve as an invaluable tool in the realm of community health nursing, offering tangible insights into the multifaceted nature of healthcare delivery within communities. These studies provide real-world examples that illuminate the complexities and challenges faced by community health nurses, as well as the innovative strategies employed to address them. Through detailed examination of specific scenarios, we gain a deeper understanding of the interplay between social determinants of health, cultural nuances, and the systemic structures that influence health outcomes.

In one illustrative case, a community health nurse working in a rural setting encounters a population with limited access to healthcare facilities. The nurse identifies a high prevalence of chronic conditions such as diabetes and hypertension, compounded by socioeconomic factors that hinder access to consistent medical care. The case underscores the importance of developing tailored interventions that not only address the immediate healthcare needs but also consider the broader social and economic barriers. By establishing mobile clinics and community health workshops, the nurse is able to bridge the gap between the community and healthcare providers, fostering a sustainable model of care that empowers residents to take charge of their health.

Another case highlights the challenges faced in urban environments, where CHNs often contend with issues such as homelessness and substance abuse. In this scenario, a nurse collaborates with local shelters and rehabilitation centers to implement a harm reduction program aimed at reducing the incidence of drug-related harm among homeless individuals. The case study demonstrates the critical role of interprofessional collaboration and the need for a holistic approach that integrates health education, counseling, and support services. Through persistent outreach and trust-building efforts, the nurse is able to facilitate access to essential health services, ultimately contributing to improved health outcomes for a marginalized population.

A third case study explores the impact of cultural beliefs on health practices within an immigrant community. Here, the community health nurse navigates the delicate balance between respecting cultural traditions and promoting evidence-based health interventions. The case illustrates the importance of cultural respect and sensitivity, as the nurse works to build rapport and trust with community members. By engaging community leaders and employing culturally appropriate health education strategies, the nurse successfully promotes preventive health practices while honoring the community's cultural heritage.

These case studies collectively highlight the dynamic and adaptive nature of community health nursing. They emphasize the necessity for nurses to be not only clinically proficient but also adept in communication, cultural respect, and advocacy. The lessons drawn from these cases underscore the critical role of CHNs in addressing health disparities and promoting equitable healthcare access across diverse populations. Through their work, CHNs not only improve individual and community health but also contribute to the broader goal of achieving health equity and social justice.

References

1. Nies MA, McEwen M. *Community/public health nursing: promoting the health of populations*. 8th ed. Elsevier; 2023.
2. Stanhope M, Lancaster J. *Public health nursing: population-centered health care in the community*. 11th ed. Elsevier; 2024.
3. Friis RH. *Essentials of environmental health*. 3rd ed. Jones & Bartlett Learning; 2018.
4. World Health Organization. Ambient (outdoor) air pollution [Internet]. 2024 [cited 2026 Feb17].Availablefrom:https://www.who.int/news-room/fact-sheets/detail/ambient-(outdoor)-air-quality-and-health
5. McDermott-Levy R, Jackman-Murphy KP, Leffers J, Cantu A. *Environmental health in nursing*. 3rd ed. Alliance of Nurses for Healthy Environment; 2023.
6. World Health Organization. Public health and environment [Internet]. 2016 [cited 2026 Feb 17]. Available from: https://www.who.int/data/gho/data/themes/public-health-and-environment
7. Aljohani K. 2024. Community health nursing in Saudi Arabia: practices and learning needs. Risk Manag Healthc Policy. 17:3239–3245. https://doi.org/10.2147/RMHP.S504277
8. Teixeira D, Nogueira M, Costa S, Amendoeira J, Martins M. Environmental health practice and quality of nursing care: a protocol for systematic review. *Online Braz J Nurs*. 2024;23:https://doi.org/10.17665/1676-4285.20246709.
9. Santos O, Melly P, Joost S, Verloo H. 2023. Climate change, environmental health, and challenges for nursing discipline. Int J Environ Res Public Health. 20(9):5682 https://doi.org/10.3390/ijerph20095682
10. World Health Organization. Environmental health Saudi Arabia 2022 country profile [Internet]. 2022 [cited 2026 Feb 17]. Available from: https://www.who.int/publications/m/item/environmental-health-sau-2022-country-profile

14 Global Perspectives in Community Health Nursing

Learning Objectives

By the end of this chapter, students will be able to:

1. Explain the concept of global health and its relevance to community health nursing, emphasizing the interconnections among biological, environmental, social, and economic determinants of health in a globalized world.
2. Identify and analyze major global health challenges, including infectious diseases, non-communicable diseases (NCDs), health inequities, climate change, and mental health issues, and evaluate their implications for nursing practice and policy.
3. Discuss the roles and contributions of international health organizations—such as the WHO, UNICEF, the World Bank, and the Global Fund—in shaping global health policies, coordinating responses to health crises, and promoting health equity.
4. Examine the functions and interrelationships of governmental, non-governmental, and multilateral organizations in addressing transnational health issues and supporting sustainable development goals (SDGs).
5. Demonstrate understanding of cross-cultural nursing principles, including cultural awareness, sensitivity, humility, and communication, and apply these principles to deliver culturally competent and equitable care in diverse communities.
6. Analyze the impact of culture and language on health beliefs, behaviors, and outcomes, and design nursing interventions that incorporate cultural values and patient-centered approaches in community settings.
7. Evaluate the development, implementation, and governance of global health policies, emphasizing their role in disease prevention, health system strengthening, and the promotion of universal health coverage (UHC).

R. I. Ashgar, *Community Health Nursing: Principles, Practices, and Perspectives*,
https://doi.org/10.1007/978-3-032-30791-0_14

8. Integrate knowledge of technological advancements and innovation (e.g., telehealth, mobile health, and digital health surveillance) to enhance global and community-level nursing interventions.
9. Critically appraise the emerging trends and future directions in community health nursing—such as sustainability, environmental health, interprofessional collaboration, and policy advocacy—and their potential to improve global population health.
10. Synthesize concepts of global health leadership and cultural competence to develop evidence-based, collaborative strategies that address global health inequities and strengthen community resilience in diverse contexts.

Global Health Challenges

In the contemporary era, global health challenges have emerged as critical concerns that demand urgent attention from health professionals, policymakers, and communities worldwide [1]. These challenges are multifaceted, encompassing a range of issues from the spread of infectious diseases to the increasing prevalence of non-communicable diseases (NCDs). The interconnectedness of the modern world, facilitated by globalization and technological advancements, has amplified the impact of these health challenges, necessitating a coordinated global response [2]. Infectious diseases continue to pose significant threats to global health, with pandemics such as COVID-19 highlighting vulnerabilities in health systems across the globe. The rapid transmission of infectious agents, facilitated by international travel and trade, underscores the importance of robust surveillance and response mechanisms. Vaccination programs, public health campaigns, and international collaborations are pivotal in controlling outbreaks and mitigating their impact on populations.

Non-communicable diseases, including heart disease, diabetes, and cancer, have emerged as leading causes of morbidity and mortality worldwide. The shift towards sedentary lifestyles, unhealthy diets, and increased tobacco and alcohol consumption have contributed to the rising burden of NCDs [3, 4]. Addressing these challenges requires comprehensive strategies that promote healthy behaviors, enhance access to healthcare services, and implement policies that discourage harmful practices.

Another pressing global health challenge is the inequity in access to healthcare services. Disparities in health outcomes are often driven by social determinants, including income, education, and geographic location [5, 6]. Vulnerable populations, particularly in low- and middle-income countries, face significant barriers to accessing essential health services. Efforts to achieve universal health coverage are crucial in bridging these gaps and ensuring that all individuals have the opportunity to attain the highest possible standard of health.

Environmental factors also play a critical role in shaping global health outcomes. Climate change, pollution, and resource depletion have profound implications for health, contributing to the spread of vector-borne diseases, respiratory illnesses, and food and water scarcity [7]. Sustainable development practices and policies that address environmental health risks are essential in safeguarding the health of current and future generations [8].

Moreover, the mental health crisis is a growing concern, exacerbated by social and economic pressures, stigma, and insufficient mental health services. The global recognition of mental health as an integral component of overall well-being is a positive step towards addressing this challenge. Efforts to destigmatize mental health issues, integrate mental health services into primary healthcare, and increase funding for mental health programs are essential in tackling this issue [9].

In addressing these global health challenges, the role of community health nursing is indispensable. Community health nurses (CHNs) are at the forefront of health promotion, disease prevention, and health education efforts. Their work in advocating for vulnerable populations, delivering culturally competent care, and fostering community resilience is vital in achieving global health goals. Collaborative efforts that involve governments, non-governmental organizations, and community stakeholders are necessary to develop and implement effective health interventions. Ultimately, addressing global health challenges requires a holistic approach that considers the complex interplay of biological, environmental, social, and economic factors. By fostering international cooperation, investing in health systems strengthening, and prioritizing health equity, the global community can work towards a healthier and more sustainable future for all.

International Health Organizations

The realm of international health organizations is vast and pivotal in shaping global health policies and initiatives. These organizations play a crucial role in addressing health challenges that transcend national boundaries, thereby promoting health equity and improving the quality of life worldwide. At the forefront of these efforts is the World Health Organization (WHO), established in 1948 as a specialized agency of the United Nations. WHO's mandate is to act as the directing and coordinating authority on international health work, providing leadership on global health matters, shaping the health research agenda, and setting norms and standards. It also offers technical support to countries and monitors health trends to ensure global health security.

Another significant player is the United Nations Children's Fund (UNICEF), which focuses on child health and welfare. UNICEF works to improve the health and nutrition of children and mothers, particularly in the most disadvantaged communities. It supports immunization programs, nutrition interventions, and water, sanitation, and hygiene (WASH) initiatives. Through its efforts, UNICEF aims to reduce child mortality rates and promote sustainable health practices.

The World Bank is also influential in the international health landscape, providing financial and technical assistance to developing countries for health-related projects. Its focus is on reducing poverty and building capacity for sustainable economic growth, with health being a critical component of its agenda. The World Bank supports health system strengthening, disease prevention, and health promotion activities, recognizing the importance of health as a driver of economic development.

The Global Fund to Fight AIDS, Tuberculosis, and Malaria is a partnership organization designed to accelerate the end of these three infectious diseases. It mobilizes and invests resources to support programs run by local experts in countries and communities most in need. By focusing on performance-based funding and country ownership, the Global Fund aims to achieve significant health impacts and foster sustainable health improvements.

Non-governmental organizations (NGOs) play a critical role in advancing international health efforts, particularly in regions where government resources are insufficient or absent. Organizations such as Doctors Without Borders provide emergency medical care in crisis settings, including conflict zones and areas affected by natural disasters. Others, like the International Medical Corps and Operation Blessing, contribute to long-term health development, disaster response, and capacity building. These NGOs often operate on the front lines, addressing urgent health needs, supporting local systems, and advocating for equitable health access. Collectively, they form a vital network of collaboration and support, each contributing distinct expertise and resources to the global health landscape. Their coordinated efforts are indispensable in responding to pressing health challenges, from infectious disease outbreaks to chronic disease management, ensuring that healthcare interventions reach even the most vulnerable and underserved populations.

Cross-Cultural Nursing Practices

Cross-cultural nursing practices are integral to community health nursing, as they emphasize the importance of understanding and respecting diverse cultural backgrounds in healthcare delivery. This approach acknowledges that cultural beliefs, values, and practices significantly influence health behaviors and outcomes [10]. Therefore, effective cross-cultural nursing requires a comprehensive understanding of cultural respect, which involves the ability to provide care that is respectful of, and responsive to, the cultural and linguistic needs of patients. A fundamental aspect of cross-cultural nursing is cultural awareness, which involves recognizing the cultural differences and similarities between healthcare providers and patients. This awareness helps nurses to avoid stereotypes and biases that can negatively impact patient care. Cultural sensitivity, on the other hand, requires nurses to be open-minded and willing to learn about different cultural practices and perspectives. This sensitivity is crucial in building trust and rapport with patients from diverse backgrounds.

Communication is a critical component of cross-cultural nursing. Language barriers often pose significant challenges in healthcare settings, leading to misunderstandings and misinterpretations. To overcome these barriers, nurses must utilize effective communication strategies, such as using interpreters or translation services, and employing non-verbal communication techniques. Additionally, understanding the cultural context of verbal and non-verbal communication can enhance the nurse-patient relationship and improve health outcomes [11].

Another important element of cross-cultural nursing is cultural assessment, which involves gathering information about a patient's cultural background, beliefs, and practices. This assessment helps nurses to tailor their care to meet the specific cultural needs of patients. It includes understanding the patient's health beliefs, dietary practices, family dynamics, and traditional healing practices. By incorporating this information into the care plan, nurses can provide holistic and culturally sensitive care.

Moreover, cross-cultural nursing practices emphasize the importance of cultural humility, which is the lifelong commitment to self-evaluation and self-critique. Cultural humility encourages nurses to recognize the limitations of their own cultural perspectives and to approach each patient encounter with an open mind and a willingness to learn. This approach fosters mutual respect and collaboration between nurses and patients, ultimately leading to better health outcomes.

Cross-cultural nursing also involves advocacy and empowerment [10]. Nurses play a crucial role in advocating for the rights and needs of patients from diverse cultural backgrounds. This includes addressing social determinants of health, such as poverty, education, and access to healthcare, which disproportionately affect minority groups. By advocating for policies and practices that promote health equity, nurses can help to reduce health disparities and improve the overall health of communities.

In practice, cross-cultural nursing requires ongoing education and training. Healthcare institutions should provide resources and opportunities for nurses to enhance their cultural respect. This includes workshops, seminars, and training programs that focus on cultural awareness, communication, and assessment skills. By investing in the cultural respect of healthcare providers, institutions can ensure that patients receive high-quality, culturally appropriate care. Overall, cross-cultural nursing practices are essential for providing effective and compassionate care in diverse communities. By embracing cultural respect, nurses can improve patient satisfaction, adherence to treatment plans, and health outcomes. The commitment to understanding and respecting cultural diversity in healthcare not only benefits patients but also enriches the nursing profession as a whole.

Global Health Policies

The intricate landscape of global health policies is a testament to the dynamic interplay of political, economic, and social forces that shape health outcomes worldwide [1]. These policies are pivotal in orchestrating international efforts to combat diseases, enhance healthcare systems, and promote public health. At their core, global health policies aim to harmonize the diverse health needs of populations with the resources and strategies available, ensuring equitable access to healthcare services across different regions. The development of global health policies is influenced by a myriad of factors, including epidemiological trends, technological advancements, and socio-political contexts [1].

Epidemiological data provide the foundation for identifying priority health issues, such as infectious diseases, non-communicable diseases, and emerging health threats. This data-driven approach allows policymakers to allocate resources efficiently and design interventions that target the most pressing health challenges. Technological advancements, on the other hand, offer innovative solutions for disease prevention, diagnosis, and treatment, thus playing a crucial role in shaping health policies. A significant aspect of global health policies is their emphasis on collaboration among countries, international organizations, and non-governmental entities. This collaborative framework is essential for addressing transnational health issues that transcend geographical boundaries, such as pandemics, climate change, and health inequities. International organizations like the World Health Organization (WHO) and the United Nations (UN) play a central role in facilitating cooperation and providing a platform for dialogue among stakeholders. Their initiatives often focus on setting global health agendas, developing guidelines, and mobilizing resources to support health programs in low- and middle-income countries. Global health policies also underscore the importance of health equity and social justice. They advocate for the reduction of health disparities by promoting universal health coverage, improving access to essential medicines, and addressing the social determinants of health. Policies are tailored to cater to the needs of marginalized and vulnerable populations, ensuring that no one is left behind in the pursuit of health and well-being. This commitment to equity is reflected in global health targets, such as the Sustainable Development Goals (SDGs), which aim to achieve universal health coverage by 2030.

Moreover, the implementation of global health policies requires robust governance structures and accountability mechanisms. Effective governance ensures that policies are translated into action, with transparent decision-making processes and stakeholder engagement. Accountability mechanisms, such as monitoring and evaluation frameworks, are crucial for assessing the impact of health interventions and identifying areas for improvement.

In conclusion, global health policies are instrumental in shaping the health landscape of the 21st century. They provide a strategic framework for addressing complex health challenges and fostering international cooperation. As the world continues to grapple with evolving health threats, the need for comprehensive and adaptive health policies becomes increasingly apparent. By prioritizing equity, collaboration, and innovation, global health policies hold the promise of improving health outcomes for all, irrespective of geographical location or socio-economic status.

Future Directions

In the evolving landscape of community health nursing, several emerging trends and future directions are poised to shape the field significantly. One of the most critical aspects is the integration of technology in health care delivery. The advent of telehealth and mobile health applications has revolutionized the way health services are provided, enabling nurses to reach underserved populations in remote areas. This technological integration not only enhances access to care but also allows for continuous monitoring and management of chronic conditions, thus improving patient outcomes [12].

Another significant direction is the emphasis on preventive care and health promotion. As the global burden of chronic diseases rises, community health nursing is increasingly focusing on preventive strategies to curb the onset of these conditions. This involves educating communities about lifestyle modifications, such as healthy eating and regular physical activity, and implementing community-wide initiatives to promote wellness [9]. Nurses are at the forefront of these efforts, acting as educators, advocates, and leaders in health promotion.

Cultural respect remains a pivotal area for future development in community health nursing. As communities become more diverse, nurses must be equipped with the skills and knowledge to provide culturally sensitive care. This involves understanding and respecting different cultural beliefs and practices related to health and illness. Future directions will likely include enhanced training programs and resources to help nurses develop these competencies, ensuring that all patients receive equitable and effective care.

The role of CHNs as policy advocates is also expected to expand. Nurses are increasingly recognized for their unique insights into the social determinants of health and are being called upon to participate in policy-making processes. By advocating for policies that address issues such as access to healthcare, education, and housing, CHNs can help to create healthier environments and reduce health disparities. Interprofessional collaboration is another area where community health nursing is expected to grow.

The complex nature of health issues today requires a coordinated approach involving various healthcare professionals. Nurses will continue to play a crucial role in these collaborative efforts, working alongside physicians, social workers, and public health professionals to deliver comprehensive care. This team-based approach not only improves patient care but also enhances job satisfaction among nurses by fostering a supportive work environment.

Sustainability and environmental health are gaining attention as important facets of community health nursing. As the impacts of climate change become more pronounced, nurses are beginning to address the health effects of environmental changes. This includes educating communities about the risks associated with climate change and advocating for policies that promote environmental sustainability. Future directions in this area will likely involve a greater focus on research and education to equip nurses with the necessary tools to address these emerging challenges [7, 8].

Lastly, the importance of mental health in community health nursing cannot be overstated. With the increasing prevalence of mental health disorders, nurses are playing a vital role in identifying, managing, and referring individuals with mental health needs. Future directions will likely see an expansion of mental health services within community settings, with nurses leading efforts to integrate mental health care into primary health services. This holistic approach ensures that mental health is given the same priority as physical health, ultimately leading to better overall health outcomes for communities.

References

1. Salm M, Ali M, Minihane M, Conrad P. 2021. Defining global health: findings from a systematic review and thematic analysis of the literature. BMJ Glob Health. 6(6):e005292 https://doi.org/10.1136/bmjgh-2021-005292
2. Edmonson C, McCarthy C, Trent-Adams S, McCain C, Marshall J. 2017. Emerging global health issues: a nurse's role. Online J Issues Nurs. 22(1):2 https://doi.org/10.3912/OJIN.Vol22No01Man02

3. Kostova D, Richter P, Van Vliet G, Mahar M, Moolenaar RL. 2021. The role of noncommunicable diseases in the pursuit of global health security. Health Secur. 19(3):288–301. https://doi.org/10.1089/hs.2020.0121
4. World Health Organization. Noncommunicable diseases [Internet]. 2025 [cited 2026 Feb 17]. Available from: https://www.who.int/health-topics/noncommunicable-diseases
5. Nies MA, McEwen M. Community/public health nursing: promoting the health of populations. 8th ed. Elsevier; 2023.
6. Stanhope M, Lancaster J. Public health nursing: population-centered health care in the community. 11th ed. Elsevier; 2024.
7. Santos O, Melly P, Joost S, Verloo H. 2023. Climate change, environmental health, and challenges for nursing discipline. Int J Environ Res Public Health. 20(9):5682 https://doi.org/10.3390/ijerph20095682
8. World Health Organization. Public health and environment [Internet]. 2016 [cited 2026 Feb 17]. Available from: https://www.who.int/data/gho/data/themes/public-health-and-environment
9. Anderson ET, McFarlane J. Community as partner: theory and practice in nursing. 8th ed. Lippincott Williams & Wilkins; 2018.
10. Leininger M. Transcultural nursing: concepts, theories, research and practice. New York: McGraw-Hill; 2002. Medical Publishing Division
11. Kim DK, Kreps GL, Singhal A. Health communication: strategies for developing global health programs. Peter Lang; 2014.
12. Badil. 2023. The role of telehealth in transforming nursing care: opportunities and challenges. Nursearcher (J Nurs Midwifery Sci). 3(02):01 https://doi.org/10.54393/nrs.v3i02.59

Epilogue

As we conclude *Community Health Nursing: Principles, Practices, and Perspectives—A Saudi Approach*, it is important to reflect on the vital and increasingly prominent role of community health nurses within the Kingdom of Saudi Arabia. Positioned at the intersection of healthcare delivery and public health, these professionals are instrumental in promoting health, preventing disease, and addressing the unique needs of diverse populations across the country.

Throughout this book, we have examined the historical, cultural, and policy contexts that have shaped community health nursing in Saudi Arabia. We have explored the principles of primary health care, chronic disease prevention, maternal and child health, epidemiological surveillance, health education, and the social determinants of health—all through a culturally grounded, locally relevant lens. The Saudi perspective is unique, shaped by rapid modernization, strong religious and social traditions, and a national vision for comprehensive healthcare reform under Vision 2030.

As the healthcare system continues to transform—toward decentralization, digital innovation, preventive care, and community empowerment—the role of community health nurses will only grow in importance. These professionals are no longer confined to clinical settings; they are educators, advocates, researchers, and agents of change within their communities. They are the link between health institutions and the people they serve, especially in reaching underserved populations, addressing health inequities, and promoting health literacy.

However, the path forward is not without challenges. Issues such as workforce development, public awareness of community health nursing roles, integration of services, and the need for localized evidence-based practices remain central to the profession's advancement. Strengthening community health nursing education, investing in continuous professional development, and fostering intersectoral collaboration are essential steps in building a robust, culturally competent, and resilient community health workforce.

In closing, this book serves not only as a guide for students and practitioners of nursing, but also as a call to action. Community health nursing in Saudi Arabia is a dynamic field, responsive to the nation's needs, rooted in its values, and committed to the health of its people. Let this work inspire continued learning, critical thinking, and compassionate service, as we collectively strive to build healthier communities and a more equitable health system for all.

R. I. Ashgar, *Community Health Nursing: Principles, Practices, and Perspectives*, https://doi.org/10.1007/978-3-032-30791-0

The manufacturer's authorised representative in the EU is Springer Nature Customer Service Centre GmbH, Europaplatz 3, 69115 Heidelberg, Germany. If you have any concerns regarding our products, please contact ProductSafety@springernature.com

Printed and bound by CPI Group (UK) Ltd, Croydon, CR0 4YY
22/10/2026
02236462-0001